RELOCALIZING HEALTH: THE FUTURE IS LOCAL, OPEN AND INDEPENDENT

RELOCALIZING HEALTH: THE FUTURE IS LOCAL, OPEN AND INDEPENDENT

www.healthrosetta.org

Published by Health Rosetta Media, Seattle, WA

This book's content significantly overlaps, updates, and expands on content published in the author's last two books, *The CEO's Guide to Restoring the American Dream* and *The Opioid Crisis Wake-Up Call ~ Health Care Is Stealing the American Dream. Here's How We Take It Back*.

This book's purpose is to shine sunlight on benefits and care models that produce world-class health outcomes while offering tools to ensure these increasingly widespread successes can be replicated in communities throughout America.

Best, Dave

Learn how the American Dream is being restored one community at a time at www.healthrosetta.org

Printed book ISBN: 978-0-9992343-6-5
E-book ISBN: 978-0-9992343-7-2

Printed in the United States of America

RELOCALIZING HEALTH: THE FUTURE IS LOCAL, OPEN AND INDEPENDENT

Dave Chase

TABLE OF CONTENTS

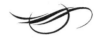

FOREWORD

Marilyn Bartlett

I've been in the business of health benefits for a long, long time now – working first for Blue Cross Blue Shield, then as a CFO for a third party administrator, and eventually serving in roles that have allowed me to make meaningful improvements in the state of Montana. If I could advise benefits professionals, employers and unions, I would say this: "You cannot settle for the status quo."

So much of this industry is shrouded in secrecy, with opaque payment systems. The money goes into the system from employers, employees, taxpayers, and consumers, who don't know what they are paying for. The system now consumes 20% of GDP, with no end to the increase in sight. We need to change this course!

The then Director of Montana's Department of Administration, Sheila Hogan, and Montana's Budget Director, Dan Villa, shared this vision and hired me as Health Care and Benefits Division Administrator to improve the state employee health plan. In that role, I used my experience and the confidence that came with it to decide the price we would pay hospitals as a multiple of Medicare, rather than simply accept the high costs the hospitals were "willing" to dish out.

Along with other measures to add efficiency, lower costs, and implement price transparency, we took a projected minus $9 million reserve balance to a positive $112 million in just over two years. Now, I'm trying to help other states do the same, much as

Dave Chase is trying to do in putting together this book.

Information on some of the very same things I did while working for the state of Montana can be found in Dave's book, specifically reference-based pricing, direct contracting, pharmacy benefits transparency, data-driven decisions, and especially value-based primary care. Dave also provides helpful insights and tips for advisors and employers to consider, from the nitty-gritty details that are needed for strong health plan design and in-depth analysis of where the money goes, to broader organizational and community efforts. Hint: It isn't over after you put the plan together. What comes next – driving organizational, community, state, and national change – is a longer-term challenge. Thankfully, it's a challenge Dave makes easier by breaking the strategies down into concrete steps.

Dave also walks local leaders, benefits advisors, and employers through the serious local, state, and national consequences they'll see if things don't change soon. Dave shows that other parts of the budget have to bend and flex and there's often not much room for that. I saw firsthand what can happen when the health care system consumes far too many tax dollars. By taking control of health care expenditures, plan design, and contracting, you can change this dynamic. We free up money for public health, primary care, and for pandemics and other unplanned disasters.

When Montana realized significant savings in the state employee health plan, the legislature retained $25 million to help balance the overall state budget *and* employees got a premium holiday. Furthermore, state employees received pay raises at the next budgeting cycle, as the health plan did not require additional funding.

More people need to see this big picture perspective and understand why we must never settle. We must never just accept something because "everyone else is doing it," and we must make the changes needed to secure a better health care system. Dave tells us how to do this and provides the support needed to move forward.

Marilyn Bartlett was selected #13 of Fortune Magazine's World's 50 Greatest Leaders of 2019 and was recently inducted into the Montana Business Hall of Fame by Montana State University. Marilyn currently serves as a Senior Policy Fellow for the National Academy of State Policy (NASHP), addressing hospital pricing.

PREFACE

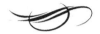

By the time I was 40, I had lost ten close friends who were my age or younger. It's a gut punch to be reminded how short our time here is, but one loss hit me harder than any other: a friend died of cancer, and the system failed her in every way. She was a talented tech executive and worked her way to the top levels of Silicon Valley. She should have had access to great health care, but got a harmful treatment plan that led to her financial, physical, and emotional ruin as her legacy to her 10-year-old daughter. It was devastating to witness.

Her death struck me particularly deeply because I realized I was part of the system. I was raised to know that if you see a wrong and don't do anything about it, you are complicit. I had started my career consulting with faith-based and children's hospitals as a revenue cycle consultant—a fancy term for generating as big a bill as possible, getting it out as fast as possible, and getting it paid as quickly as possible. At one time, this was simply to ensure that a hospital didn't forget to bill for something, but it became the root of a scheme that is arbitrary, abusive, and has absolutely devastated the working and middle class in America. Like my friend before her death, hundreds of thousands of victims of our corrupt health care system file for bankruptcy every year—even though 70% of them have insurance. I saw the fear in my friend's eyes thinking about her daughter's future, knowing that even after working hard and being extremely successful, she wasn't going to be able to leave her with much, if anything.

Not long before my friend's passing, I had been leading the most successful technology platform in health care. I was excited about how patients and doctors could finally realize value from easy-to-use software after decades of mainframe computers. But despite breakthrough technologies that could improve patient outcomes, that's not what hospitals wanted to buy. All they wanted were systems tuned to game every reimbursement opportunity the industry had to offer. Despite being at the top of my game in health care, I couldn't be party to that and vowed I wasn't going to work on technology that I knew was going to do more harm than good. I was frustrated that I didn't have the solution, so I left health care for over a decade.

Around the time I was returning to health care, a high school kid asked me to buy a candy bar for her school fundraiser. Great, I said, were they raising money for a band trip? No. It turned out they were raising money for science lab supplies. What?! Taxes paid for that stuff when I was a kid.

Turns out this often isn't the case anymore, primarily because of health care. Bill Gates devoted an entire TED talk to how health care has been devastating education: larger class sizes, laid off teachers, fewer music and arts classes, and increased college tuition for state universities and community colleges. He also outlined how devastated education budgets would impact the future by preventing bold experiments and limiting opportunities for excellence. When Gates gave his talk, California alone owed more than $60 billion in health benefits costs that it couldn't pay. I started my K-12 education in California at a time when the state was generally considered to have the best education system in the country; today it has the lowest high school graduation rates in the entire country—and the highest student to teacher ratio.

The scale of the financial and medical devastation that health care has wrought on America is something most people can't imagine. Financially, health care's hyperinflation has driven more than two decades of wage stagnation and decline. Today, 60% of the workforce makes $20/hour or less, while health insurance premiums for a family of four are over $20,000 per year.

With over half of the workforce having a deductible greater than $1,000, most Americans are a bad stubbed toe away from financial ruin. And these are the people who have insurance!

For example, even as the country focuses on the COVID-19 pandemic, we continue to grapple with an older massive public health crisis, the opioid crisis, which is a self-inflicted wound driven almost entirely by a dysfunctional health care system. While in Boston last fall, not far from "Methadone Mile," I saw two things that we now know are profoundly connected—gleaming billion-dollar medical towers and students "on strike" because of school underfunding.

Believe it or not, we can go a long way to stopping the opioid crisis in its tracks, while fixing education underfunding and preventing or better preparing the country for future crises, through access to great, value-based primary care, a critical foundation for a fair, rational, affordable, and effective health care system.

I've found real hope in the solutions I've discovered. Every structural solution to prevent what happened to my friend and countless others has already been invented and proven, and is working someplace in this country. A small hotel company has the best benefits package of any employer I've ever seen—and they spend 55% less than employers of similar size. In addition to providing quality, affordable health care to employees and their families, they've invested a small fraction of what they saved into the local community and school system, which are seeing stunning results: crime has gone down by 67% and high school graduation rates have doubled to essentially 100%. It sounds unbelievable, but it's true, and it's happening in Orlando right now.

The most amazing discovery I've made in studying successful innovations is that the best way to slash costs is to improve health benefits and outcomes. How could I not share this great news?

The excitement from health care professionals, elected officials, employers, and other civic-minded Americans is contagious. If you've picked up this book, you are part of the solution.

No matter who or where you are, you can join this effort to catalyze change and restore both hope and health to the community where you live and work.

There is no time to lose, especially after seeing how badly undermined primary care and poor public health infrastructure made the U.S. much more vulnerable to COVID-19. Fortunately, there are many things you can do to prevent further dysfunction.

For example, work to ensure that your company, union, or community has access to great primary care. Join the Health Rosetta community to share your successes and learn from those of others. If you are a city leader who makes health care-related decisions, lead by example with city employees and use your bully pulpit to reinvent health care in your community. If you are a union leader, follow the example of dozens of school districts around the Pittsburgh area, where labor and management leaders put aside old differences to work together for benefits that boost the health—and bottom line—of all parties.

Also, write down every organization you have influence over and share with them that the best way to slash health care costs is to improve health benefits. Share this book with them— we've made a free download available of it and my past books, such as *The CEO's Guide to Restoring the American Dream*, at www.healthrosetta.org/friends. We care more about spreading success than losing a few book sales.

Whatever your role, start with one organization and one tactic. For too long we've let health care crush the American Dream. We cannot take another 20 years of economic depression for the working and middle class. Whether we know it or not, we all contributed to this mess. Now, it's on us to fix it. When change happens community by community, it is impossible to stop. Yes, health care stole the American Dream. But, it's absolutely possible to take it back. Join us to make it happen in your community.

To learn more, read on or visit healthrosetta.org. What is the Health Rosetta? The blueprint for evidence-based health purchasing. It's a practical approach built on what successful purchasers do.

For ongoing insight, best practices, and updates, subscribe to the Health Rosetta newsletter at healthrosetta.org/employers. Throughout the book, you will find a variety of email addresses where you can send information related to chapters and become part of the solution. However, if you have success stories of how communities are being rebuilt, or have general ideas or feedback, email me at dave.chase@ healthrosetta.org.

Preface

INTRODUCTION

If you want to get to the root cause of an issue, just ask, "Why?" That's what I do every time I see employees strike, and usually the answer – no matter the industry – is, at least in part, "health care." A few recent examples:

In the auto industry, in the longest strike between GM and the United Auto Workers (UAW) union since 1970,[1] the UAW fought to protect hourly workers' 3% health care cost share, while also arguing for better wages, job security, and other benefits.[2]

In education, the Dedham (Massachusetts) Education Association struck—the state's first strike in 12 years[3] —to get the Dedham School Committee to reduce teachers' health insurance contributions.[4]

And in the health care industry itself, the University of California (UC) Service and Patient Care Technical Workers (part of the American Federation of State, County and Municipal Employees Local 3299) struck the university, arguing that UC is outsourcing work to people they pay less and refusing to increase wages for existing workers.[5]

That last example may not, on the surface, seem to be a direct response to health care cost concerns. However, health care spending is the underlying issue here too.

Employers have had to dedicate an increasingly significant part of their budget to health care costs each year. As a result, many have compensated by cutting into other parts of the budget – like wages, retirement benefits, etc. – or forcing employees to bear more of that cost burden via high-deductible health plans. Still others, like UC allegedly, have outsourced functions to remove the cost burden of health benefits, which increases the number of working poor who are employed by contractors that do not offer insurance and who cannot afford publicly available health insurance.

The truth is, the public sector could do more to make their health plans more affordable for all people. It could also improve outcomes in their communities if local dollars weren't being swallowed up by, in many cases frivolous, projects like the $1 billion expansion of Massachusetts General Hospital.[6] Hospital leaders' edifice complex often takes large sums of public and/or private dollars away from sectors and initiatives that truly matter for the sole purpose of producing a shiny new building for people to admire—a building whose revenue is dependent on the public's unfortunate need to visit it.

In Texas, health care dollars could be better used in attempting to reduce the state's obesity rate – it's the 10th highest in the country[7] – by addressing food deserts, improving school lunches, and funding primary care that includes health coaching. Or, the state might follow the superior health care model Pittsburgh-area schools used to ensure smaller class sizes and better teacher pay and benefits.

Understanding how we can free up health care dollars to accomplish these goals, or really any goals that are important to states, is what this book sets out to do. It walks readers through how much money is wasted on our current catastrophic health care system at the national level, the state level, and even the employer level. It further explains how that catastrophic system has given birth to subsequent public health crises – the example I'll use here is the opioid crisis – and how we allowed this to happen. Finally, it points the way for us to end the current system by designing low-cost, high-quality, parent-approved Health plans.

We're spending more than enough money to get the best health care system in the world. In places, we actually already have it – and not just for the rich. The only real question is whether we can massively replicate what we already know works beautifully. My dad passed away from Parkinson's last year, and I can honestly say that I don't know of any model in the world that could have exceeded the care he received through his Health Rosetta-type health plan. As a country, we can easily afford to implement this model as it's much less costly than the disaster that is our status quo health system.

Changing the world starts with changing health care's status quo, and to do that all of us must first rally together. There are many inspiring responses to the COVID-19 pandemic. We have seen actions taken in 10 days or weeks that might have taken 10 years under ordinary circumstances. I am counting on you to rise to the challenge to drive change in whatever sphere you have influence. With this book as your guide, I encourage you to go forth and continue to push forward the health care revolution that's gaining more and more momentum each and every day.

Health care isn't expensive. What is expensive is profiteering, price-gouging and edifice complexes that prioritize building Taj Mahals over disaster readiness. After all, only $0.27 of every $1 ostensibly spent on health care goes to the primary value-creators – nurses, physicians and other clinicians.

Introduction

A WORD ABOUT WORDS

Health care always seems to use ten different words for essentially the same thing, each with some supposed slight variation in meaning that isn't even consistently used by those of us in the industry. I have also included terms that may be unfamiliar to those outside the health benefits profession. To minimize confusion, I have tried to use consistent terminology, as follows.

- **Benefits broker, consultant, and advisor.** These three terms are often used interchangeably in the real world to refer to people who arrange, negotiate, and/or purchase a health plan on behalf of a third party. I use broker to signify a person who operates under the status quo, taking a highly conflicted approach to purchasing health benefits. I use advisor or consultant to signify someone operating under the modern, high-value, transparent approach.
- **ERISA.** The Employee Retirement Income Security Act of 1974 is a federal law that sets minimum standards for most voluntarily established pension and health plans in private industry to provide protection for individuals in these plans.
- **Fully insured.** This is the common but misleading term for health plans provided by traditional insurance carriers. We prefer the term "carrier controlled." For employers, there is little doubt that if an organization has a "bad

year" the carrier will claw back whatever they may have lost in that one year and more than make up for it in future years-as if the prior "good years" had not provided ample reserves. Also, 70% of medical bankruptcies are filed by "fully insured" people.

- **Health plan.** This refers to a specific health benefits plan, whether fully insured or self-insured.
- **Insurance company or carrier.** These refer to the organizations that provide insurance and/or self-insured plan administration services
- **PBM.** Pharmacy Benefit Manager is a Third-Party Administrator (TPA) of prescription drug programs for commercial health plans, self-insured employer plans, Medicare Part D plans, the Federal Employees Health Benefits Program, and state government employee plans.
- **People.** I use a couple of different terms depending on context. Individual is the default. Patient is for people receiving care. Member or employee refer to individuals from a health plan or employer's perspective.
- **Plan administrator.** This is the organization that performs the noninsurance pieces of a health plan, like claims adjudication. It includes Administrative Services Organizations (ASO) tied to insurance companies and independent Third-Party Administrators (TPA).
- **Provider organization and clinician.** These terms cover the people and entities that provide health care services. This includes physicians, nurses, hospitals, health systems, and other providers of health care services.
- **Quadruple Aim.** Refers to the simultaneous pursuit of improving the care team experience (both professional and non-professional members of the care team), the patient experience of care, improving the health of populations, and reducing the per capita cost of health care.
- **Self-insured or self-funded.** These are organizations, typically with more than 100 employees, that may use an insurance company provider network, but pay the

claims and take on the financial risk themselves. We prefer the term "employer-controlled health plans" as there is outside insurance (stop loss coverage) in most cases. Only enormous organizations may be entirely self-insured

- **Stop-Loss Insurance.** All but the largest employers have stop loss policies that cover unpredictable claims such as cancer, organ transplants and other outlier claims.
- **TPA -Third-Party Administrators.** Self-insured organizations normally use an independent third party to administer health claims. A variant of this is Administrative Services Only (ASO) organizations that are owned by insurance carriers with resulting pros and cons laid out in Part III.
- **Workplace wellness program.** The term wellness has been co-opted by a large industry of vendors that largely sells products with no or negative return on investment (ROI). I use this more specific term to refer to these programs.

CHAPTER 1

THE FUTURE OF HEALTH WILL BE LOCAL, OPEN, AND INDEPENDENT

It should come as no surprise that the most successful solutions to society's most challenging problems do not now and will not in the future arrive with the cavalry from Washington, D.C. After all, the great societal challenges that America has been tackling over the last several decades – civil rights, energy independence, climate change, better food – all have been fueled from the bottom up.

This is certainly true when it comes to health care: an industry that spends more on lobbying than oil and gas, defense, and financial services *combined* is going to have its way with Congress.[8] I've taken to calling most D.C. politicos "preservatives" rather than progressives or conservatives, as they get paid to preserve the status quo. The fact remains that over the last couple of decades neither Democrats nor Republicans have accomplished much to address the two biggest failings of the U.S. health care system: pricing failure and overtreatment. At the same time, government's failed approaches created collateral damage including under-resourced public health infrastructure.

Health care is particularly suited to a bottom-up approach because it begins at home. The fundamental value creation in health care is the relationship between an individual and his or her care team. The more intermediaries and bureaucrats that get inserted into that relationship, the greater the chance for value to be extracted rather than added.

Chris Brookfield has close to 20 years' experience designing networks and services that empower people in emerging markets both in the U.S and abroad. In 2004, he left mainstream venture capital to focus on investments with broader and more beneficial human impact. He and his team played an instrumental role in lifting tens of millions of people out of poverty through microfinance, small business loans, rural hospital development, and slum improvement finance in India. He is now applying his systems change model to remaking the U.S. food system as well as new services for the next era of capitalism.

Tired political labels get swept aside when people come together to solve their issues. Brookfield's work in food has revealed a natural collaboration between farmers and those in the local food movement, even though farmers tend to be more politically conservative and local food people tend to be more politically progressive. We find the same thing in health care, where free market-oriented, conservative physicians are pursuing the same objectives and using similar tactics as progressive union leaders.

Models that deliver systemic change, says Brookfield, have three big themes in common: They're local, open, and independent. In this chapter, I'm going to show how health care can capitalize on these same themes using excerpts from Brookfield's paper on system change (shown in italics).

Local

Focusing on local [reveals] a number of intrinsic advantages [that] are often overlooked [in the larger picture]. First, by decreasing scale, solutions can appear to problems that seem too complicated to solve at the global scale. For instance, re-engineering the food system or decreasing poverty really are intractable when viewed at the global scale. Even the basic atoms of these systems — people — are invisible. By dialing into local, new features and relationships emerge.

In their new book *The New Localism*, urban experts Bruce Katz and Jeremy Nowak describe a diversity of needs at the local level. They compare cities such as Detroit, which may need to demolish blighted housing to boost value, to hot-market cities such as Boston, which may need to build and preserve more housing to meet demand. State and federal legislatures tend to enact one-size-fits-all solutions and, often for political reasons, prefer spreading public resources evenly, despite widely varying needs. New localism allows communities to focus on the challenges they actually have rather than on the national issue "du jour."

Localism realigns entrenched politics. It's striking how new alliances are formed at the local level that are impossible at the national level — where conservatives see new federalism, independence, entrepreneurism, and local business, and progressives see community building, health, nutrition, education, and nurturing. In health care, individuals receive care from local clinicians, yet only $0.27 of every dollar spent goes to these locally based, value-creating clinicians. Between $0.50 and $0.75 of every dollar goes to the drug supply chain, health systems, and health plans that are usually headquartered elsewhere. This is at the heart of how the "sick care" industry has extracted resources that would otherwise go to social determinants of health that are fundamentally local (e.g., schools and social services). The table below shows where the health care dollar goes.

~$0.45	Fraud	Extractive or no value
	Misdiagnosis & overtreatment	
	(High-cost, massive overtreatment: spinal & stent procedures; high misdiagnosis areas: oncology, musculoskeletal, etc., ranging from 25%-67%)	
	Abusive & arbitrarily high prices	
	(Massive pricing failure: prices for similar quality often vary 2-10x)	
~$0.30	Insurer or health system administration & overhead	Often extractive
~$0.25	Paying high-value care providers	Generally not extractive

Table 1: The Distribution of a Health Care Dollar

Note: These are very high-level approximations for illustrative purposes. They're based on multiple, widely recognized sources and generally accepted data, including PwC's "The price of excess– identifying waste in health care spending" and the Institute of Medicine's[9] estimate of waste at 30%-50% of spending. Other data points are outlined elsewhere in the book, including rates of misdiagnosis and pricing failure.

One of the key architects of the Patient Protection and Affordable Care Act (ACA), Bob Kocher, MD, echoes this reality in a *Wall Street Journal* op-ed entitled "How I Was Wrong about Obamacare,"[10] in which he outlines the importance of independent, locally controlled medical practices:

Personal relationships of the kind found in smaller practices are the key to the practice of medicine. Small, independent practices know their patients better than any large health system ever can ... [They] are able to change their care models in weeks and rapidly learn how to use data to drive savings and quality ... [I]t does not take [them] years to root out waste, rewire referrals to providers who charge less but deliver more, and redesign schedules so patients can see their doctors more often to avert emergency-room visits and readmissions.

I believed then that the consolidation of doctors into larger physician groups was inevitable and desirable under the ACA. What I know now, though, is that having every provider in health care 'owned' by a single organization is more likely to be a barrier to better care.

Open

Openness is an advantage, largely because information networks have coalesced over the past 15 years and have exponentially increased the flow of information to local communities. There is no way to transmit proprietary ideas at anywhere near the speed and coverage that open-sourced ideas move.

Openness is proving itself in an array of settings. The beer market is mature and has been dominated in the U.S. by a couple of behemoths, yet craft brewers recently have grabbed 24%[11] of beer spending. How? Craft brewers are radically open with each other regarding how to succeed, recognizing that their real competition is the mega brewers, not each other.

One of the failings of the wildly underperforming status quo health care system is how poorly insights and breakthroughs get disseminated. Research shows that it takes 17 years for effective breakthroughs to become mainstream.[12] Therefore, a central tenet of the Health Rosetta is to create an open, Wikipedia-like "hive mind," which makes it much easier to understand and deploy approaches that sustainably outperform traditional approaches to Quadruple Aim objectives.

Near the conclusion of a great new book, *Our Towns*, James Fallows echoes the theme of taking what's already working and sharing it much more broadly. He quotes Philip Zelikow, a professor at the University of Virginia who said to Fallows:

"In scores of ways, Americans are figuring out how to take advantage of the opportunities of this era, often through bypassing or ignoring the dismal national conversation. There are a lot of more positive narratives out there – but they're lonely, and disconnected. It would make a difference to join them together, as a chorus that has a melody."

Katz and Nowak describe a new circuitry of civic innovation in which innovative practices are adapted from one city to another – cities in radically different circumstances that are simultaneously trying to solve similar challenges. The adaptation of solutions is accelerated by new city-related associations that share innovation, industry-specific organizations such as the Health Rosetta, or major foundations such as the Rockefeller Foundation.

Independent

As with scale, we are hybridizing our approach to system design [of next-generation wheat mills] to incorporate the best of both local and conglomerated infrastructure. By integrating business models with existing social movements, we achieve network connectivity beyond the local watershed, allowing the sharing of resources, information, and values. By allowing each of these businesses to function autonomously within this fabric and grow to their fullest individual potential, an individual mill can utilize the control and hierarchical scalability typified by corporation[s] ... [A]t the same time, the fabric as a whole achieves quick responses, flexibility, and adaptability – responses [that] are inhibited by corporate concentration.

The first broad application of the local, open, and independent model is the vanguard benefits advisors, who are the torchbearers of the next health era. Perhaps no job is more underestimated in all of health care in terms of its potential to help (or hurt) the working and middle class of America. Our experience has been that the vast majority of employers defer most of their health benefits decision-making to their benefits broker, a different animal altogether. As outlined elsewhere in the book, this is often to the detriment of employers and their stakeholders, whether they be employees, shareholders, taxpayers, or otherwise.

The Health Rosetta benefits advisors are building the next generation health economy by replicating what is proving successful in a wide array of settings: public and private employers, rural and urban areas, large and small employers. Again, replication is the key word.

Given that the primary value creation in health care is fundamentally a local endeavor tuned to local dynamics, we believe replication is the way change will happen. This is a fundamental contrast to massive top-down, large-scale programs. Replication varies from application to application; scalability seeks to apply the same things everywhere. This distinction is subtle but absolutely critical to achieving success.

Post-Political

One indicator that a movement is ready for development in the commercial sphere is ... when [it] ceases to be perceived as political within the relevant communities. While movements remain politicized, there is insufficient agreement; when the community itself is split in its support, this method of commercial development is doomed at the outset. On the other hand, it was obvious in the case of both microcredit and local food that virtually everyone in the local communities agreed with the underlying premise. When community business models and commercial values align, they were able to attract nearly unanimous support.

As Katz and Nowak point out, new localism is also nonpartisan and powerful.

"The regular engagement of business, civic, and academic leaders elevates pragmatic thinking and commonsense discourse and crowds out the inflammatory rhetoric associated with partisanship and ideology. New localism is intensely focused on maximizing value for long-term prosperity rather than short-term private profit or political gain. Cities' main message to the federal government today is 'first, do no harm.'

"Millions of decisions are made by subnational leaders and ordinary citizens, and these decisions build communities, drive economies, educate children, catalyze innovation, and change lives. New localism is both representative of and restorative of the democratic ideals and principles on which the republic was founded and which sustain Americans in good and bad times."

Perhaps it is time to dust off the public referenda process to garner support for transformative investments in the future. A great example of this is how the Austin electorate voted to tax itself during an economic downturn in order to fund the Dell Medical School. Central to the mission of the new medical school is serving as the community health care provider. Even in the short time since they opened, they've tackled previously resistant problems. For example, the working poor in Austin had an 18-month wait to be seen for orthopedic issues. Today, it's down to about a week, thanks to on-the-ground problem-solving versus simply pouring more resources into a clearly flawed approach.

The Original Sin

In *An American Sickness*, Elisabeth Rosenthal explained how the way we structured health insurance was in some ways the original sin that catalyzed the evolution of today's medical-industrial complex. This doesn't mean health insurance is a bad thing. It means health insurance as we have known it is a bad thing. We need to re-do health insurance to support the health care system we want, not the one we've got. Brookfield believes that huge risk pools are the heart of the problem.

When local networks are scaled up, you add hierarchy, says Brookfield, and this creates an opportunity for theft and redirection. Brookfield's genius has been understanding how social missions can be nested within free markets and how local control is a path to broad, positive change. This has been applied to microcredit, rural hospital development, and more. He has a proven track record of bipartisan approaches to tackling extremely difficult problems such as systemic poverty, lack of access to health care, and a food production system that has harmed local economies while producing subpar food. The following is Brookfield's reaction to Rosenthal's comment:

All group risk pools – health insurance, life insurance, credit insurance, disaster/property insurance – have a long social history. They all evolved out of village/community mutual aid groupings. So, for instance, along with microcredit (which has analogs that go back thousands of years) there were all kinds of group risk insurance. The community would pay if one member had an unanticipated tragedy.

These semiautonomous systems work very well at the community level. They are efficient and well supervised by their own participants. In this kind of network – some call it a fabric – there is much mutual overlap: walls are thin, and gossip travels fast, which drives the [development of] community governance. This kind of signaling among community participants is really highly effective at reining in [systemic] abuses, as well as bureaucracy, lag times, and translation errors. This is the essence of Elinor Ostrom's insight that won her the Nobel Prize for economics. But these systems go completely haywire when 'scaled up,' which creates opportunity for theft and redirection.

Persuading individuals to buy insurance is kind of backwards. I saw this in India all the time. Individuals do not value their own risks – their relatives and neighbors do. We could not get individuals to buy insurance. We made buying life insurance compulsory to receiving a much bigger benefit – personal loans. Then we quickly sold 10 million policies. It would be good for American policy makers to be reminded that insurance is not an attractive sale to an individual; the beneficiaries of insurance, fundamentally, are the family, community members, and invested financial institutions, not the insured.

Most modern insurance vastly scales up the number of people who bear the burden and, in the process, adds enormous cost while losing effective oversight. Pools of more than 1,000 people are redundant and may reduce resilience, as the ballooning overheads outweigh the marginal benefit from wider risk sharing. Pools of hundreds of thousands or more people simply mean more power and money for the administrators, plus hugely expanded costs for end-of-life interventions that are a huge burden for smaller pools. Bigger scale + more cost = additional costs from providers ... and on we turn.

For nearly all people nearly all of the time, says Brookfield, we would be better off with community risk pools, self-governed, for nearly all our risks, using traditional pools only as reinsurance.

The primary issue of outlier claims is easily addressed. Over 100 million Americans are in self-insured plans. All but the largest have stop-loss policies for outlier claims. This allows companies as small as 20 people to self-insure without risk of financial ruin if they have an unfortunate medical incident.

'Buy Local' Programs Will Reinvigorate Communities

Increasingly, communities realize the value of "buy local" programs that increase community resilience and economic opportunity. Today, the vast majority of communities send a large amount of money to out-of-town bureaucracies to pay for services that are mostly delivered locally. It's quite odd if you pause and think about it. In contrast, the Rosen Hotels case study is a microcosm of how a community can be literally transformed (crime down, high school graduations up, etc.) by reinvesting money that would otherwise have been squandered on giant out-of-town bureaucracies. Likewise, Pittsburgh has shown how a local insurance pool can ensure that education budgets no longer get eviscerated by a wasteful health care system.

Even in countries perceived to have centralized health care systems, ownership and administration is pushed down to much more local levels. Communities like Jönköping, Sweden have been internationally recognized for how they innovate and "real-locate" monies to fit the needs of community members. Jönköping leaders are aware that clinical health care drives less than 20% of health outcomes, so balancing that spending with investments in clean air and water, better schools, job training, and other opportunity creation maximizes community well-being.[13]

In many ways, we already have this today in a variety of communities, from employers (self-insured and captive) to unions to health-sharing ministries. Health Rosetta co-founder Sean Schantzen tells me all the time about ways organizations hedge their bets against risks of all kinds, many of which are extraordinarily complex and unpredictable. For example, the wide range of reinsurance products, commodities options, currency hedging, etc. are all forms of insurance that enable organizations to tailor their protection to their comfort level with risk.

We know that our current approach to health insurance isn't well-received. Customer satisfaction with status quo health insurance is lower than virtually any other sector of the economy. The beauty of the approach Brookfield articulates is the blend of local control and accountability with the scale advantage from appropriate use of technology and modern business tools. Without local accountability, distant bureaucracies are vulnerable to abuse. Consequently, a cascade of stifling bureaucracy gets layered on to the point we've reached today, where an alphabet soup of MACRA, MIP, MU, PCMH, HCAHPS and more crushes our nurses and doctors. People sometimes conflate re-localizing health care and health insurance with past clumsy efforts to pool risk, many of which haven't worked.

They didn't work for the following reasons:

- They brought organizations together that had no connection or local accountability and were driven by distant state bureaucracies.
- They were predicated on buying from out-of-area intermediaries and insurance or provider companies versus locally controlled provider organizations. With that came all the baggage outlined in other parts of this book, such as PPO networks that once made sense but have become value-extractors from local families and economies. Case studies throughout this book of unions, employers, and

municipalities demonstrate how they are more effective than insurance companies at slashing health costs by managing things at an appropriate scale. Why? They have aligned interests absent from most intermediary arrangements in health care.

- They used the same old health payment approaches that have proven to deliver mediocre health outcomes, eat up extraordinary sums of money, and make clinicians' lives miserable. Hardly a recipe for success. When social missions are nested within free markets and local control, there is a path to broad, positive change that is embraced by people who put their humanity before tired political labels.

In the hopes of ensuring that you and your organization don't likewise experience failure, the next chapter digs into how to produce high-quality, low-cost, and even parent-approved health plans.

Key Takeaways and Things to Think About:

- By decreasing scale to a local level, solutions can appear to problems that seem too complicated to solve at the global scale.
- Roughly half of every dollar spent on health care adds no value; much of it is extracted out of local economies to out-of-town health plans, health systems, and investors, even though health care is fundamentally local. The value-creating nurses and doctors receive only $0.27 of every dollar ostensibly spent on health care.
- There is no way to transmit proprietary ideas at anywhere near the speed and coverage that open-sourced ideas move. The arc of health bends toward openness.
- Transforming health care requires re-doing health insurance to support the health care system we want, not the one we've got. This doesn't mean health insurance is a

bad thing. It means health insurance as we have known it has created a multitude of perverse incentives that harm both patients and clinicians.

- Combining the best of local autonomy with the benefits of modern financial and technology infrastructure can be achieved in post-political movements.

CHAPTER 2

HEALTHCARE IS BREAKING LOCAL, STATE, AND FEDERAL BUDGETS

In September, Marty Makary, a professor at Johns Hopkins and author of *The Price We Pay: What Broke American Health Care – and How to Fix It*, published an op-ed in *USA Today* revealing how many federal dollars the healthcare-cost beast is consuming. According to his Johns Hopkins colleagues, it is eating nearly half (48%), which includes funding for Medicare, Medicaid, Social Security, military health benefits, health benefits for federal employees and their dependents, plus interest.[14]

Our federal government spends 48% of its money on health care and still health care devastates state budgets all across this country, with serious consequences we're already seeing in public health and education.

Sadly, it was bloated health care spending that did more to devastate public health funding than anything else. Consequently, thin public health investments left the country woefully unprepared for the COVID-19 pandemic, making it far worse than it needed to be.

In the meantime, high-quality schools and programs are being washed away, the collateral damage ranging from larger class sizes and fewer arts programs to teacher layoffs and increased college tuition. None of these casualties are good for kids or the nation's future.

Fortunately, there is a better way (see the case study on Pittsburgh [Allegheny County] Schools in the last chapter of this book), but let's first understand the magnitude of the problem.

Health Care's Hyperinflation Is Breaking U.S. Schools

Bill Gates gave a TED Talk[15] on the macro view of the impact of state budgeting on education. Gates looked at data from California, but it's not a problem unique to California. At the time of this talk, only $3 million had been set aside for retiree benefits, whereas $62 billion had been committed.

It's bad today but will only get worse over time as health care continues to consume an increasing proportion of states' budgets. And if we don't solve education funding on a sustainable basis, we're only putting a Band-Aid on a growing, gaping wound.

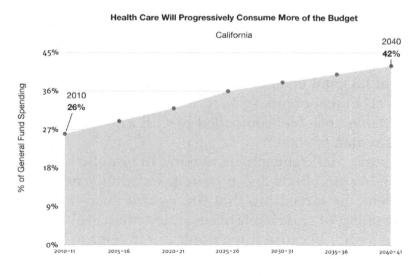

Figure 1: Slide from Bill Gates's TED Talk, "How State Budgets Are Breaking US Schools"

15

Proof that we have yet to really address the underlying issue here – health care – is the fact that we still lurch from one education-funding crisis to another. That's because even in states such as Massachusetts that pass legislation to pay teachers more, guess what? Teachers don't take home one more dime, because every new dollar allocated to teacher salaries gets eaten up by health care costs.

Massachusetts is actually a cautionary tale for the rest of the country. While there are pockets of brilliance in the state's health care system that demonstrate its potential – such as its response to the Boston Marathon bombing – overall the system is clearly out of control: literally in the shadow of billion-dollar medical towers you'll find ground zero for the Massachusetts opioid crisis, dubbed "Methadone Mile."

Unlike public health crises such as polio and HIV, the opioid crisis is a logical and tragic byproduct of our health care system (more on that in Chapter 4). But that's not the only way our catastrophic health care system has devastated and enraged communities. As health care has stolen from education, Boston students felt compelled to go on strike to protest lack of funding[16] despite a robust economy. Billions have supported hospitals' edifice complex (e.g., Massachusetts General Hospital's plan for another billion-dollar medical tower despite a current excess of hospital beds) instead of addressing things like high lead levels in school pipes.[17] In fact, Massachusetts hospitals are so profitable, they feel compelled to shift $1.6 billion in profits to the Cayman Islands.[18]

In sum, Massachusetts is making the implicit decision to increase hospital beds and pursue tax shelter schemes rather than focus on something that drives true health – stopping the poisoning of children. This is an imbalance all states must work to avoid, because if we don't put an end to it, as Gates points out, it will only get worse, making the dreams we have to improve schools – bold experiments, measuring teacher effectiveness, providing incentives for excellence – impossible to achieve.

We don't have to look far to see just how bad it will be. The slide below shows the impact of health care starving other spending at the state level.

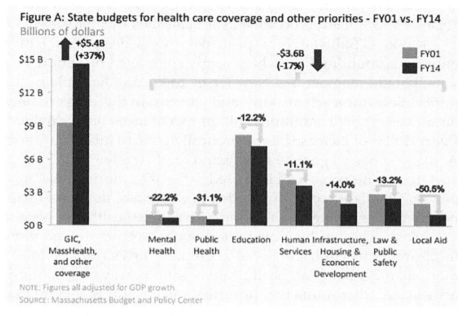

Figure A: State budgets for health care coverage and other priorities - FY01 vs. FY14

NOTE: Figures all adjusted for GDP growth
SOURCE: Massachusetts Budget and Policy Center

Figure 2: Health Policy Commission, "List of Figures in 2013 Cost Trends Report by the Health Policy Commission."[19]

If you look at the above items that have been cut, they are the ones that drive health outcomes more than clinical care.[20] The result? For the first time in our country's history, lifespan has flattened.[21] Just as bad, the quality of life has suffered. Ten years ago, I can't remember seeing one of those mobility scooters and now they are everywhere.

A Local Case Study

ProPublica's Marshall Allen recently exposed how New Jersey's health plan for school employees pays out-of-network providers virtually whatever they want. Dozens of acupuncturists and physical therapists earned more than $200,000 in 2018 from school staff alone.[22] One brought in $1 million. As one clinic put it, "We strategically target schools and municipalities where there are self-funded plans, where we as a company can continue to grow." As outlined later, carriers administering teachers' money are happy to enable "blank-check" claims processing to facilitate their own profits.

Kevin O'Sullivan is a principal (non-CPA partner) in a national accounting firm who recently completed his tenure as a school board member in a New Jersey town, and he explains the implications for teachers, kids, and citizens. In the 15 years since he moved to his community, his property taxes have doubled. Every dollar of increase has theoretically gone to fund education. Actually, it has all gone to feed health care's waste.[23]

If our lifespans had increased 50%-100% during that time period, we might accept that trade-off. Obviously, that hasn't happened. We are paying Cadillac prices for a Pinto health care system.

Worse, during this time period, we've seen more and more local programs cut back. Because property taxes can't be raised more than 2% per year, health care is eating away at school priorities and other municipal priorities such as infrastructure that provide us with clean air, clean water, and more.

As O'Sullivan explains in a letter to the editor of a local paper, the impact on taxes is obvious:[24]

"Let's extrapolate the expense drivers in the budget. If salaries go up 2% per year, at $750,000, and health care goes up 15% each year, call it $1.5 million, we are looking at an increase of $2.25 million per year, every year.

"If we can only raise taxes $1.1 million, we need to cut $1.15 million each year. The takeaway here is that health care expenses alone are going up faster than we can raise taxes.

"This is not opinion. It is fact.

"In 2009, the premium for a family plan was $13,200. This year (2014), it will cost $28,000. That is a 112% increase over five years.

"It has taken up $4 million more in expense [in] our budget. This $4 million obligation now threatens even the continuation of existing programs for our students and hampers the ability to invest in new programs. We are paying more taxes and getting fewer services. This is not sustainable."

Teacher Unions Must Step Around to the Other Side of the Table

Nothing jeopardizes school funding and teacher salaries more than health care costs; anyone with a primary school education can see that health care's hyperinflation "tax" is starving our retirement savings and gutting education.[25] The old models of school boards and teacher unions duking it out have failed, but both parties share a common interest in wanting the best education for our kids while fairly compensating our beloved teachers. Clearly, the boards and unions should join in common cause to do a reset on the health care status quo in their communities.

A district typically pays approximately $20,000 per staff member for health benefits, factoring in dependents. This buying power is enough in and of itself, but it is feasible for districts to join forces with other large public and private sector employers in their community to command even more.

Framework: Health Rosetta Components

Sourced from real-life successes of employers everywhere. Collectively, the components sustainably reduces health care spending by 30-40% or more.

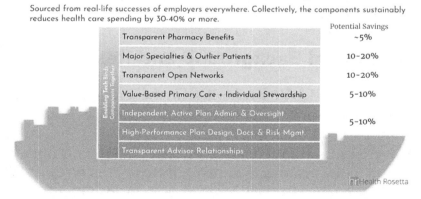

	Potential Savings
Transparent Pharmacy Benefits	~5%
Major Specialties & Outlier Patients	10–20%
Transparent Open Networks	10–20%
Value-Based Primary Care + Individual Stewardship	5–10%
Independent, Active Plan Admin. & Oversight	5–10%
High-Performance Plan Design, Docs. & Risk Mgmt.	
Transparent Advisor Relationships	

Figure 3: "The Health Rosetta."[26]

Fortunately, all of the structural models necessary to fix health care have already been invented, deployed, proven, and modestly replicated. Few have brought them together in one place like we've done with the Health Rosetta framework (see below), but when it happens the results are breathtaking, opening the door to a new era of economic development.

Key Takeaways and Things to Think About:

- The health care system itself has become the greatest immediate threat to our freedom to pursue health and the American Dream.
- Health care has redistributed virtually all salary increases from employees to an underperforming health care system over the last 20 years, creating an economic depression for the working and middle class.
- Health care is choking funding for public health, education, public infrastructure, and social services.
- Transforming health care requires re-doing health insurance to support the health care system we want, not the one we've got. This doesn't mean health insurance is a bad thing. It means health insurance as we have known it has created a multitude of perverse incentives that harm both patients and clinicians.

Additional Background and Resources:

- What You Don't Know About the Pressures and Constraints Facing Insurance Executives Costs You Dearly [https://bit.ly/2NfQnwp]
- 7 Tricks used to redistribute money from your organization to the healthcare industry [https://bit. ly/30JWIYN]
- PPO Networks Deliver Value – And Other Flawed Assumptions That Crush Your Budget [https://bit. ly/2Y7Jh3i]

CHAPTER 3

ECONOMIC DEVELOPMENT 3.0: COMMUNITIES TAKE CENTER STAGE

In his book *The Coming Jobs War*, Jim Clifton, Chairman of Gallup, makes a strong case that the United States is already in World War III. Unlike the previous wars, which dictated which countries would lead the world in prosperity as a function of property, the current war will dictate which communities will prosper by winning the lion's share of jobs. Civic leaders can and should seize this opportunity to reinvent their communities and build infrastructure.

The wisest leaders will shift how their communities think about economic development. It turns out that having a high-value health ecosystem is likely to be of greater benefit than a tax break. Conversely, communities with expensive health care have what amounts to a large health care tax, which will push businesses away or, at a minimum, impair their bottom line and the well-being of their workforce.

The Post-Copernican View

Economic Development 1.0 was largely a function of geography: successful towns emerged near ocean and river ports or along transportation routes and capitalized on the need to shift goods and people efficiently.

Economic Development 2.0 has been largely a function of marketing: communities throw tax breaks at corporations to attract or retain them without always considering the long-term effects. For example, building hospitals was perceived as an economic driver despite considerable evidence that adding capacity is an economic drainer after the "caffeine hit" of initial construction. This pre-Copernican view of health care puts hospitals and medical technology at the center of the health universe. The post-Copernican view puts individual and community well-being at the center of a properly functioning health ecosystem.

Unfortunately, Italy learned the hard way. *The New England Journal of Medicine* highlighted a study on the hazards of having hospitals rather than homes and community-based clinics as the front-line of a battle against a pandemic. The report stated "[H]ospitals might be the main COVID-19 carriers, as they are rapidly populated by infected patients, facilitating transmission to uninfected patients.[27] Pandemic solutions are required for the entire population, not only for hospitals." Just as centralized military communication systems were vulnerable to nuclear attacks (and thus the Internet was developed to maintain communication even if there was a nuclear hit), an outdated "mainframe" model of health care delivery left many countries more vulnerable. Centering on hospitals, rather than care at home, public health and primary care was a key contributor to outbreaks worsening.

Economic Development 3.0 recognizes that all the tax breaks in the world are dwarfed by whether a community has a high-value or low-value health ecosystem. After payroll, health benefits are often the largest cost for most employers in both the public and private sectors. Just as manufacturers shift production to low-cost manufacturing centers, employers will be attracted to high-value health communities. For instance, IBM is making decisions on where to locate new technology centers based on the health care value equation. Such decisions represent thousands of jobs for communities vying for growth opportunities.

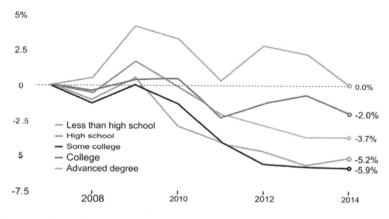

Cumulative percent change in real average hourly wages, by education, 2007-2014

Note : Sample based on all workes age 18-64.

Source: Epl analysis of Current Population Survey Outgoing Rotation Group microdata

Figure 4: 2014 Continues a 35-Year Trend of Broad-Based Wage Stagnation.[28]

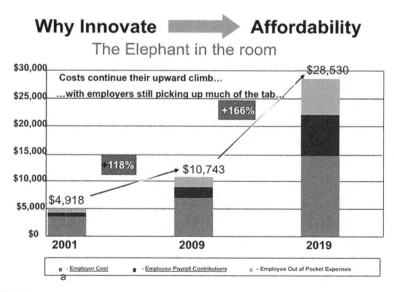

Figure 5: Per capita spending for IBM employees 2001, 2009 with projection for 2019.[29]

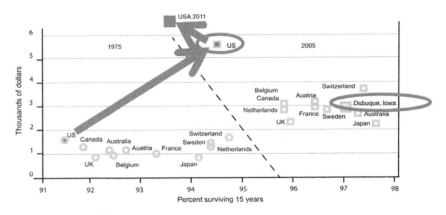

Figure 6: Per capita spending and longevity by country, 1975 to 2005, by locale.

As we have seen, employers foot most of the health care tab[30] and are starting to flex their muscles. Thus, IBM shifted from thinking about health benefits as a soft benefit to seeing them as a major supply chain input that will impact its profitability. The company decided where to locate 4,000 new hires based on their analysis of where they would receive the best value from their health care expenditure. After looking at the graph above, it's easy to understand why they picked Dubuque, Iowa.

Given the wide cost differentials, CFOs and CEOs are failing in their fiduciary responsibility if they do not move to modern health care delivery models that are proven to save money while maintaining or improving health outcomes and patient satisfaction. This is a scary prospect for communities that have high-cost health care with average outcomes.

Winston Churchill was quoted as saying, "Healthy citizens are the greatest asset any country can have." It stands to reason that we should measure that asset. One could imagine a Community Well-Being Balance Sheet as a leading economic indicator of prosperity. On the asset side of the ledger would be things like clean air, clean water, the number of high school/college graduates, community centers, and so on. On the liability side would be things like a Superfund site or outstanding hospital bonds.

We could also imagine something like a Gross Community Product: the collective revenues generated by local businesses subtracting out health care spending as a measure of people who are not able to contribute to community well-being. Forward-looking economists are developing new economic indicators to better reflect the health of communities.

Taxation without Representation

Jeff Brenner, MD, founder and long-time executive director of the Camden Coalition of Healthcare Providers, currently senior vice president of Integrated Health and Social Services at UnitedHealthcare Community & State, and a 2013 MacArthur Genius Grant recipient, spoke about health care as a tax on a community[31] that the residents didn't get to vote on – a tax that negatively affects a community's competitiveness. He points to a "giant hospital bond market" that brought too many hospital beds online. An empty hospital bed, says Brenner, is the most dangerous thing in America.

"In the center of New Jersey ... a couple years ago, they built two ... $1 billion hospitals, 10 miles apart, very close to Princeton. One is called Capital Health, and the other is Princeton Medical Center. I don't remember anyone in New Jersey voting to build two brand-new hospitals. But we are all going to be paying for that the rest of our lives. We'll pay for it in increased rates for health insurance. And, boy, you better worry if you go to one of those emergency rooms, because the chances of being admitted to the hospital when there are empty beds upstairs ... are ... much, much higher than when all the beds are full – whether there's medical necessity or you need it or not. I'd be very worried if you live in Princeton that there are now two $1 billion hospitals waiting to be filled by you."

Every health system CEO I've spoken with agrees with health policy expert Paul Keckley, Ph.D., that there is at least a 40% over-capacity of hospital beds,[32] yet some communities are still building.

A recent Harvard School of Public Health study of 195 hospital closings found that the closures had no discernible impact on outcomes.[33] In fact, in countries that have shifted from a "sick care" model to a model that is focused on health and well-being, more than half of hospital beds were no longer needed. This is something to celebrate. While we must be mindful of short-term impacts on individuals working in these facilities, there are higher and better uses for most of these people (e.g., health coaches and investments in health-enhancing infrastructure).

Even though many health systems are tax-exempt nonprofits, perverse incentives have created a dynamic where revenue growth has become a central objective. In reality, tax-exempt nonprofits make up 70% of the most profitable hospitals,[34] perhaps because their boards are typically made up of business leaders who reflexively view revenue growth as the goal when it should be community well-being and addressing major issues such as the opioid crisis. Hospital executives also realize it's easier to justify enormous compensation packages if their institution is generating massive revenue increases every year. As Axios reported, "Large not-for-profit hospital systems now resemble and act like Fortune 500 companies instead of the charities they were often built as. They consequently hold immense financial and political power."[35]

In contrast, forward-looking nonprofits focus on longterm economic sustainability and their mission to serve as stewards of community health. With all the changes in health care, it's just a matter of time before more enlightened boards fundamentally rethink their mission to emphasize the 80% of nonclinical factors that contribute to health and well-being.

Closing a Hospital Opens Other Doors

One of the most respected health care leaders in the country, David Feinberg, MD, formerly the CEO of the renowned Geisinger Health System, believed his "job ultimately is to close every one of our hospitals," in order to take care of individuals at home, work, and school.

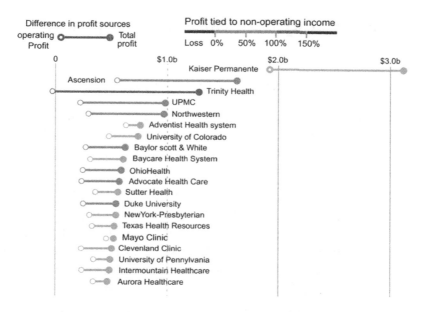

Figure 7: Herman, Bob, "Hospitals Are Making a Fortune on Wall Street."

As overcapacity gives way to hospitals optimized for the health of communities, those communities will realize a bonus: hospitals are often in locations with high real estate values. According to David Friend, chief transformation officer at the consulting firm BDO in Boston, "A hospital could be worth more dead than alive."[36] Hospitals are often in city centers with great access to transit. Wide hallways, thick walls, and high ceilings make them easy to convert to housing. Communities have repurposed hospitals to a wide variety of uses, from low-income senior housing to health and wellness centers to office space.[37]

Being alarmed by a hospital closing is understandable. However, experience shows that this can open great opportunities while rarely affecting health outcomes. Naturally, ensuring sufficient ER/ICU capacity should be viewed as an investment in public health versus a profit or referral center. An analogy from military bases is enlightening: the closing of Philadelphia's naval shipyard was bitterly fought, yet now the repurposed naval yard is the most dynamic development in Philadelphia.[38]

Rethinking Economic Development

Here are some examples of how forward-looking civic leaders are embracing Economic Development 3.0:

- Freeing up financial resources formerly dedicated to unnecessary and harmful clinical procedures allowed Rosen Hotels & Resorts to invest heavily in its community; the result was a reduction in crime of 67% and a doubling of high school graduation rates. The Rosen case study outlines how a single private employer pulled this off, but any employer – public or private, large or small, corporate or government – can do the same. In New Jersey, public and private unions joined with a Democratic Party-dominated legislature and then-governor Chris Christie to find common ground around improving health benefits to lower health care costs.
- Communities have found that "Shop Local" programs lead to more dollars circulating in the local economy. Health care is a fundamentally local interaction, yet the value creators (nurses and doctors) receive $0.27 of every dollar spent, with a much larger percentage going to bloated administration or overhead, fraud, waste, and abuse that robs communities. Municipalities as employers and trendsetters are increasingly contracting directly for health services in order to keep money in the community. For example, directly contracting with locally owned surgery and imaging centers[39] rather than with health system chains owned by outof-towners is increasingly common. The potential to recirculate dollars with locally owned health care provider organizations is enormous.
- Mayors and economic development directors are catalyzing locally controlled health insurance pools referred to as "captives," where multiple organizations pool risk. Think of it as the health insurance equivalent of the Green Bay Packers, which is owned by a community with local con-

trol but can tap into national-scale contracts, reinsurance, and technology.

- As large employers themselves, municipalities are getting much smarter about how they purchase health benefits, using the components outlined in the Health Rosetta blueprint. With respected organizations such as PwC acknowledging that more than half of health care spending is waste, it is logical that financially strapped municipalities are rethinking their approach, as Kirkland, Washington, and Milwaukee, WI have demonstrated. (See case studies in Chapter 11.)

- The historically adversarial relationship between school boards and teacher unions has hurt communities throughout the country. Proactive city leaders recognize healthy schools are one of the most important factors in attracting and retaining citizens. In an announcement about a new teachers' union agreement in a school district that covers one of the wealthiest areas of the country, one major accomplishment cited was that "teachers will see protection from rising health care costs," largely as a result of school district concessions. While this is laudable, the smartest districts and unions are realizing they're on the same side when it comes to health care costs and can collaborate to slay the health-care-cost beast, as they did in Pittsburgh. (See the Pittsburgh case study in the back of the book for more).

Sooner rather than later, we can expect other developments along the same 3.0 spectrum. Cities will incorporate true health needs into master planning and review building permit applications with a deep understanding that health care is a supply-driven market. The more supply there is, the more demand will increase with little regard for value and community well-being. Approving more health care build-out virtually guarantees a massive burden on local citizens. Just as some communities have zoning to limit big box retailers, one can imagine zoning that recognizes the drain more big box hospitals can put on a community.

Forward-looking city attorneys and state attorneys general will challenge the noncompete agreements that doctors have signed as being against the public interest. In particular, primary care physicians (PCPs) are foundational to a more effective health system. Though they were ostensibly money losers in the waning fee-for-service industry, PCPs can refer more than $8 million per year in revenue to the rest of a health care system. As a result, health systems have gobbled them up to protect their flank and create captive referral channels, insisting on anti-competitive deals that harm a well-functioning health ecosystem.

Key Takeaways and Things to Think About:

- Economic Development 3.0 recognizes that all the tax breaks in the world are dwarfed by whether a community has a high-value or low-value health ecosystem.
- Closing a hospital can open doors to myriad economic benefits to a community. Transforming hospitals and hospital beds to higher and better purposes is a sign of progress.
- "Shop Local" applied to health care provides an unprecedented economic stimulus opportunity.

CHAPTER 4

HEALTH CARE IS STEALING MILLENNIALS' FUTURE, BUT THEY WILL TAKE IT BACK

If we can't slay the health care beast, millennials will see their future stolen from them. As the largest generation in history and now the largest chunk of the workforce (see Figure 8), they will make their presence felt.

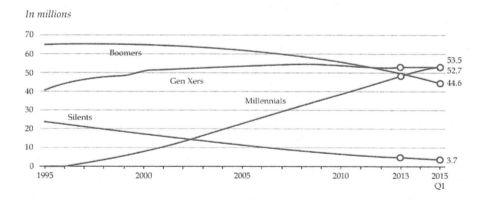

Figure 8: Richard Fry, "Millennials Surpass Gen Xers as the Largest Generation in U.S. Labor Force," Pew Research Center, (July 4, 2016).[40]

Whether through government favoring the largest special interest groups (e.g., hospitals, pharmaceutical companies, and insurance companies) rather than the people or through self-in-flicted mistakes (e.g., the HMO "gatekeeper" and denial of care debacle), health care has been remarkably resistant to forces try-ing to disrupt it for decades – forces that have driven change in virtually every other sector from financial services to retail to travel. Millennials will bring this disruption to health care.

Becky and Her Biggest Expense

An influential book I read is David Goldhill's *Catastrophic Care: Why Everything We Think We Know about Health Care Is Wrong*. Goldhill is co-founder and CEO of Sesame, an online marketplace for discounted health services serving uninsured patients and other direct-pay customers, and chair of the board of directors of the Leapfrog Group, an independent national employer-spon-sored organization focused on hospital and medical safety. But in 2009, he was CEO of The Game Show Network when he lost his father to a hospital-acquired infection, complicated by numerous errors. This experience caused him to bring his financial acumen to bear on health care instead.

If he didn't break it down with well-sourced figures, Gold-hill's conclusions would be unbelievable. Who could imagine that during their adult lives, one out of every two dollars earned by millennials will go to a health care system that is the polar opposite of what they want and value? If, that is, the current tra-jectory is not altered. Keep in mind that while well over 80% of health-related spending goes to the "sick care" system, which only drives 20% of health outcomes.

Figure 9 tells a terrifying story, but more shocking is how conservative the assumptions behind the numbers are. The nar-rative of Becky that follows is drawn from Goldhill's book.

Share of Lifetime Earnings of a Millennial That Will Go to Health Care Unless We Change Course

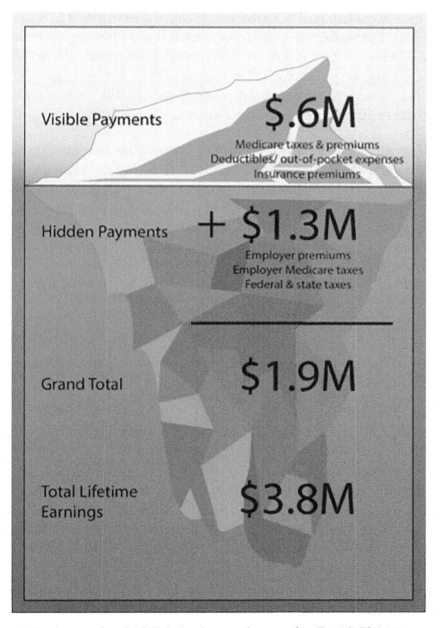

Visible Payments — $.6M
Medicare taxes & premiums
Deductibles/ out-of-pocket expenses
Insurance premiums

Hidden Payments — + $1.3M
Employer premiums
Employer Medicare taxes
Federal & state taxes

Grand Total — $1.9M

Total Lifetime Earnings — $3.8M

Figure 9: Numbers come from Goldhill's book and are over the course of a millennial's lifetime.[41]

Let's give this millennial a name, Becky, and make a few assumptions about her life. We'll say she gets married at 30 and has two children. She works until she's 65 and dies at 80. We will also assume her income grows every year by 4%, so that at retirement she is earning $180,000 a year. To simplify the analysis, we'll have Becky's husband leave her to join an ashram when he turns 65, so she's only responsible for her own Medicare premiums. Let us also give Becky a stroke of good fortune and say that she and her dependents stay healthy, with no major health crisis requiring large out-of-pocket expenditures.

Now, allow me to make a truly crazy assumption just for the sake of argument. Let's assume that health care costs grow at only 2% a year – half of Becky's income growth. This hasn't been true for 45 years, but we can always hope. Given all those factors, how much do you think Becky will contribute to the health care system for herself and her dependents over her lifetime? I'll give you a hint: Becky will earn $3.85 million over her career. The answer is $1.9 million! If she has a working spouse, the two will contribute $2.5 million into this system over their lifetimes.

How has this happened? Remember that Becky is almost certainly unaware of how many ways she is paying into the health care system, even though she'll probably put more into that system than she spends on anything else over her entire life.

This projection takes on added urgency when you consider that obesity rates have tripled among young adults in the past three decades, from 8% in 1971-1974 to 24% in 2005-2006, thanks to the diet of what Michael Pollan calls "food-like substances" that their boomer parents fed them.[42] This is causing millennials to engage more broadly in the health care system much earlier than previous generations. As Figure 10 shows, only 20% of health outcomes are the result of clinical care. The areas that represent the other 80% are a good place to start to understand where millennials will likely take our health care system.

Finally, the jig is up. A do-it-yourself health reform movement is rising – and not a moment too soon. Solutions are coming from the edges: from forward-looking employers, innovative towns, fed-up physicians, and, especially, from millennials wising up. Ask any venture capitalist whom they study to get insight into the future, and they'll give you a clear answer – millennials.

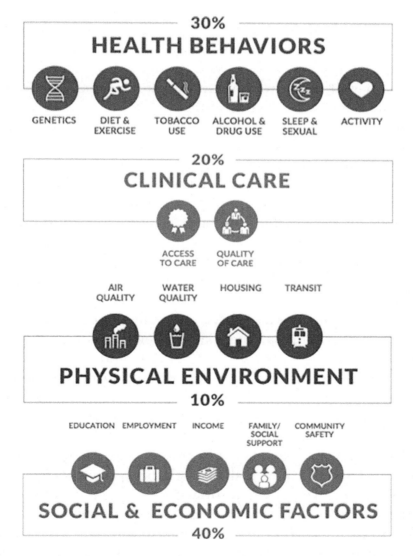

Figure 10: In the future, the health ecosystem will focus on the true drivers of outcomes, of which clinical care is only 20%.[43]

Millennials to the Rescue

Millennials, people 24-39 in 2020,[44] have driven society-wide change in many areas. Their early adoption of technology made smartphones, social media, and services such as Uber pervasive across all generations. That row of empty storefronts in your town? That's the power of millennials.

Financial services are a good example of millennials steering the market away from today's market leaders.[45] Wellknown brand strategist Adam Hanft, author of *The Stunning Evolution of Millennials: They've Become the Ben Franklin Generation*, could have been talking about health care when he wrote:

"[Millennials'] faith in technology is understandable. Algorithms don't act in their own self-interest. Algorithms weren't responsible for dreaming up subprime loans and nearly bringing down the financial system. Millennials didn't trust authority and conventional sources of wisdom before the meltdown. Imagine now. Wealthfront argues that millennials: '... have been nickel-and-dimed through a wide variety of services, and they value simple, transparent, lowcost services.'"[46]

"Millennials have also driven the growth of Wealthfront, an alternative to traditional financial advisers who frequently steer clients toward their own firm's financial products. In contrast, Wealthfront has mimicked, in algorithmic form, the portfolio investment strategies of the most sophisticated wealth managers (e.g., rebalancing portfolios, tax-loss harvesting), traditionally available only to very high net worth individuals."

Hanft goes on to offer a word of warning to the financial industry that could just as easily be applied to the health care industry: "The giants of financial service haven't seen the [volcanic] shifts that travel, media, entertainment and home thermostats have. They will. Depending on who you are, the Ben Franklin generation is composed of 80 million Benedict Arnolds." Industry giants may want to ignore this trend, but millennials are the canary in the coal mine because the fact is everyone wants these features. As Danny Chrichton, a venture capitalist investor at CRV – and a millennial – has said, "Consumers want to be able to manage their finances from their phones and tablets while limiting their visits to bank branches and bank tellers. Plus, everyone hates bank fees, particularly their complexity and lack of transparency. The difference is that millennials are willing to shop elsewhere, because we are simply not going to accept that these are the only products on the market."[47]

Another example of millennials forcing change is the newspaper industry. Millennials ignored newspapers as a source of news but also as the de facto place to buy/sell items. (Craigslist anyone?) Undermining classified ads, which were roughly half of newspaper profits, made newspapers a demonstrably worse product. Those profits previously supported the reporting that has declined sharply over the last 10 years. Many papers have even had to eliminate editions on some days, further accelerating the trend.

Health Care Priorities: Cost and Convenience

The health-system parallels to newspaper classified ads are profit centers such as cardiac catheterization labs – sometimes nicknamed "cash labs," as they are also centers of overuse. Cardiac catheterization led to the development of wonderful interventions – angioplasty, coronary artery bypass grafts, stents – that revolutionized cardiology in the 20th century. Without question, this saved lives. But the fact that these procedures are grossly overused is no longer in question either.

Overuse in health care is not simply a matter of wasted resources, money, and time. It exposes patients to terrible harm – often including death. Here's what happened to one 52-year-old woman who came into an ER with chest pain after starting a new exercise regime. Shannon Brownlee, senior vice president of the Lown Institute, described the situation at the Health Care Town Hall Meeting at the Frontier Cafe in Brunswick, Maine, on Nov. 6, 2014:

"The emergency doctor thought it was almost certainly a pulled muscle, but just to be sure he ordered a new and special CT scan of the heart. It showed a little something, as these scans so often do, and so just to be sure he sent her to the cath lab. There was nothing wrong with her heart until they perforated her aorta. They did an emergency bypass from which she recovered; but then she had graft bypass rejection and she had to have her heart replaced. This is a person who came into the emergency room with a pulled muscle."

Cath labs are no longer the sound investment they once were. Millennials, more than previous generations, want to know all the diagnostic and treatment possibilities when they're sick or injured and are more likely to select lower-cost, less-invasive treatment options. This is also what most people of all generations want when given full information. Again, millennials are just the drivers.

Given their insistence on new ways of doing business on every front, it's not surprising that millennials are avoiding the ill-designed norms in health care – for example, selecting a doctor. It's not that millennials aren't loyal to their physicians when convenient, but they're far more willing than boomers to "doctor shop" until they are satisfied. They're looking for same-day appointments, online scheduling, easy access to their medical records, and the option to text or email the doctor between visits, according to KQED's Chrissy Farr.[48]

Most people who use ZocDoc – a website that helps individuals schedule doctor's visits, some of them on the weekends and in the evening – are millennials. And in addition to convenient scheduling, many ZocDoc doctors use convenient methods of communication, like text or email, to talk to patients.

Retail clinics, typically found in national pharmacy chains like Walgreens and CVS, are another innovation being embraced by cost and convenience-conscious millennials. The number of retail clinics in the United States grew from 200 to 1,800 between 2006 and 2014, while visits grew sevenfold to 1.5 million.[49]

A PNC health care survey found that 34% of people ages 18 to 34 prefer retail clinics – about double the rate of 17% for baby boomers and 15% for older seniors.[50]

New Benefits Choices for Smart Communities

Millennials may be more interested than their parents in getting the most for their health care dollar, but nearly three in four of them are confused about their benefit options, according to a 2016 Harris Poll. And almost half would rather clean out their email than research those options.[51]

Why is this important to you or your client's company? Because that same survey shows that 76% of millennials say health care benefits strongly factor in their decision about where to work.[52]

Millennials are now the biggest portion of the workforce and will be 75% of it in 2025.[53] The time has come for benefits brokers to fulfill their promise and guide their clients toward developing new benefits programs optimized for millennials.

For example, smart employers can shift their workforce to a higher-performing benefits package through tiers that introduce changes. Under this strategy, the old "get less, pay more" status quo package becomes "Tier 2." The new benefits offering is "Tier 1" and is the default package for new employees.

Freelancers now make up 35% of U.S. workers and collectively earned $1 trillion in 2016.[54] That translates to 55 million people. While these aren't all millennials, the newly named CEO of the Amazon – Berkshire Hathaway – JP Morgan Chase health organization spoke to the imperative to fill this need. During an interview with PBS's Judy Woodruff, Dr. Atul Gawande stated:[55]

"Tying how you get your health care to your place of employment is going to become less and less tenable as fewer and fewer people are getting coverage through employment. We miss this important statistic … Over the last 10 years (data was from 2005-2015), 94% of net new job growth was in forms of employment that had no health care benefits. It was alternative work forms. It was gig employment, independent contracting, temporary workers. That's the world my kids are now walking into. When they get their employment, they are most likely to be in that category."

Gawande, of course, was speaking even before the COVID-19 pandemic highlighted the perilous nature of health insurance tied to your employment.

As outlined in Chapter 2, forward-looking mayors are embracing the Economic Development 3.0 mindset. Increasingly, millennials are choosing where they want to work geographically, before they choose the specific company or job they'll choose. Mayors, such as Lauren Poe of Gainesville, Florida, are actively working to make their communities more attractive by ensuring there are great health benefits options that go beyond typical ACA plans, which leave many people are functionally uninsured at a time when the majority of U.S. households have less than $1,000 in savings. This is because, if you have a bronze or silver plan, the average deductible is $5,873 and $3,937 respectively.[56] In other words, even while technically being insured, you are a bad stubbed toe away from financial ruin.

This is the millennials' moment. They're not alone, but they will suffer the devastating consequences of an out-of-control health care system more than anyone. When millennials rise to the occasion, I believe they will be remembered as the Greatest Generation of the 21st century.

I also believe in the enormous potential of community-driven change from the bottom up. Central governments have largely reached the limits of what they can achieve. Increasingly, community-level change is where the action is.

The good news is that slaying the health care cost beast is straightforward, as I explain in my TED Talk[57] and as the case studies in the last chapter of this book demonstrate.

Paradoxically, the best way to slash health care costs is to improve health benefits. The effects are far-reaching, improving whole communities and working to solve one of the greatest public health crises of this century: the opioid crisis.

Key Takeaways and Things to Think About:

- On the current path, millennials would become indentured servants to the health care system, spending half to two-thirds of lifetime earnings on health care. Millennials will ensure that never happens – in the process driving tremendous change in health benefits unlike we have ever seen.
- We all ultimately desire what millennials desire, whether it's smartphones, better food, social media, or better health care.
- As health care change will happen in phases, millennials are natural early adopters of greatly improved health care.

CHAPTER 5

THE OPIOID CRISIS ISN'T AN ANOMALY

For 37 years, Tom L. Shupe, a senior manager at an Oklahoma manufacturer, has been on the frontlines of the challenges facing U.S. manufacturing. He's full of insights, but the most surprising one is that he blames substance abuse – specifically opioids – for most of these challenges. "It's all addiction issues," says Shupe. He calls the opioid crisis, which is really an epidemic of addiction, "probably the biggest threat in manufacturing, period."[58]

Here is something even more shocking: Employers are unwitting accomplices, enablers, as well as victims. From 1999 to 2017, more than 477,000 people have died from an opioid overdose.[59] Overwhelmingly, those suffering from opioid use disorders are working age people or their dependents. Through our health benefits, we have funded a self-inflicted wound that is emblematic of the even broader dysfunction pervasive in our health care system.

The COVID-19 pandemic has exacerbated the issue with overdose up 42% year or year.[60]

Let's look at just one example. A major challenge of physically demanding, hourly jobs is that if you don't work, you don't get paid. Sixty percent of the workforce makes $20 per hour or less[61] – many of them paid hourly. When an injury occurs, the worker must choose between not working, and not getting paid, or continuing to work despite the pain.

Opioids start as a short-term fix, enabling the worker to stay on the job, but they also slow – and can even prevent – healing.

If the worker has the predisposition to addiction, a vicious escalating cycle takes off. Jordan Barbour, director of clinical operations, psychiatry, and addiction medicine at Geisinger Health, described the common progression from addiction to work issues to job loss to street drugs, incarceration, and Hepatitis C, all costing the family and community dearly.

Beyond the obvious human toll, there is a financial imperative to solve this crisis. Supporting early identification of addiction, along with access to effective treatment and relapse prevention, doesn't just help the sick and suffering. It makes great economic sense.

Make no mistake; The opioid crisis is a complicated issue over 30 years in the making. But companies have played a major role in creating and sustaining the crisis. And a vanguard of employers are realizing that they have a major role to play in solving it, and that the solutions fall well beyond what the government alone can do.

In this, the epidemic is a microcosm and mirror of our failing health care system as a whole; ending it will move us meaningfully down the path toward solving the larger crisis.

NOTE: There is a growing trend that equates people suffering from chronic pain with people suffering from opioid addiction. In fact, there is an array of rare diseases, such as Ehlers–Danlos syndrome, where well-managed opioid regimens can be the appropriate course of treatment. We must be careful that the zeal to address opioid abuse doesn't inflict unnecessary suffering on those with chronic pain. This is where having adequate time to treat patients as individuals is imperative; other countries manage to work with these long-term patients without triggering an opioid crisis.

A Weight Around Employers' Necks

Before delving into the antidotes, let's take a quick look at the damage opioids are wreaking on the American economy in general and employers in particular.

Here's a good starting point: Opioid overdoses – often in conjunction with other central nervous system depressant drugs like benzodiazepines or alcohol – are now the leading cause of death for working people under 50 years old, surpassing deaths from guns and car crashes.[62]

LinkedIn's Work in Progress podcast looked at the negative impact of the opioid crisis on employers.[63] There were a couple big takeaways:

- At a Congressional hearing focused on opioids and their economic consequences, Ohio Attorney General Mike DeWine estimated that 40% of job applicants in the state either failed or refused a drug test.[64] The result: In certain places, solid middle-class jobs can't be filled. In Congressional testimony in July 2017, then Federal Reserve Chair Janet Yellen connected opioid use to a decline in the labor participation rate.
- The issue is amplifying labor shortages in industries like trucking, which has had difficulty for the last six years finding qualified workers. It's also pushing employers to broaden their job searches, recruiting people from greater distances. The issue is not just workplace safety and productivity, but whether workplaces need humans at all. Some manufacturers claim opioids are forcing them to automate faster.

Some may find drug testing intrusive, but many jobs – whether in manufacturing or other sectors such as transportation – pose potentially huge consequences from accidents. You may not recall that opioids were to blame for the Staten Island Ferry disaster that killed 11 and injured scores.[65] A very big problem for employers is "presenteeism," where an employee performs sub-optimally, often as a result of impairing

pain or medications, especially opioids. Unlike cocaine or heroin, where a confirmatory drug screen results in termination, a "legitimate" prescription for oxycodone and Xanax is a much murkier problem.

The New York Times reported that when workers who strained their backs received higher doses of opioid painkillers than their coworkers in a similar predicament, they had a tendency to stay off the job three times longer.[66] In addition, it reported that when insurer Accident Fund Holdings reviewed its claims, it found that "when medical care and disability payments are combined, the cost of a workplace injury is nine times higher when a strong narcotic like OxyContin is used ... The sum of an employee's medical expenses and lost wage payments – was about $13,000. But when a worker was prescribed a short-acting painkiller like Percocet, that figure tripled to $39,000 and tripled again to $117,000 when a stronger, longer-acting opioid like OxyContin was prescribed."

In that same article, Dr. Bernyce M. Peplowski, the medical director of the State Compensation Insurance Fund of California, said that insurers' policy of covering painkillers but not evidence-based physical therapy approaches "have created a monster."

It's Not Just Opioids

Cathryn Jakobson Ramin devoted an entire book (*Crooked: Outwitting the Back Pain Industry and Getting on the Road to Recovery*) to how little evidence informs our back pain industry. And opioids aren't the only class of medication that is being inappropriately prescribed. The depressant benzodiazepine – think Ativan, Klonopin, Valium, Xanax, and other such "benzos" – is as well.

In fact, prescriptions for these drugs – often used to combat anxiety, seizures, and insomnia – more than tripled from 1996 to 2013. Worse, fatal overdoses increased more than four times during the same time period.[67] Considering that benzodiazepine is the go-to psychiatric medication[68] and the No. 1 most-prescribed U.S. medication, this isn't all that surprising. Why they're prescribed is puzzling though: there's little evidence that they work, plus they aren't supposed to be used for long periods of time.[69]

Recently, I was sharing with a neighbor of mine the mess we have created with opioids. She confided in me that she is dependent on benzos. She is the CEO of a rapidly growing, young company and hit a tough spot a couple of years ago. Her doctor prescribed benzos to address her anxiety without giving her any idea of how addictive they can be nor what the plan was to wean her off. She is extremely angry and frustrated now, knowing how difficult it is to wean off. She can't stop her life as a mother and business owner for 30 days or longer to wean herself off and feels trapped. A frequent statement you read is that withdrawals from benzos are worse than heroin. As one put it, "Benzos withdrawal can kill you.[70] Heroin withdrawal just makes you wish you were dead."

Sadly, the exploding benzos crisis demonstrates how the opioid crisis isn't an anomaly. It *is* our health care system.

The Path Forward

While we must be smarter about treating those already afflicted with opioid addiction, we must also turn off the spigot to clean up the mess. The silver lining of the opioid crisis is that it shines a light on just how abysmally our health care system has been performing. True health starts at home and in our communities, not in hospitals or in pills.

At the end of Sam Quinones's gripping book on the opioid crisis, *Dreamland*, he argues that the sustainable fix is "a community that addresses social determinants of health like safe neighborhoods, quality jobs, and a health care system that can treat those afflicted with opioid use disorders while preventing others from being drawn into the hell of addiction." Employers using the opioid crisis as a catalyst to change their approach to health care can do a great service by revitalizing the broader community. By extension, a growing employer then has a better pool of prospective employees to draw on.

Put simply, employers who adopt Health Rosetta-type benefits programs are far more likely to have much lower rates of employees and dependents suffering from opiate use disorders. Given that the opioid crisis isn't an outlier situation but a microcosm of a larger dysfunction, it's clear how solving one of the largest public health crises in American history can serve as a catalyst for dramatically improving our entire health care system.

Now, let's look at the 12 drivers of the opioid crisis, understanding how this crisis came to be, and then how we can best solve it.

NOTE: The vast majority of doctors, even those who are salaried employees, have no financial incentive to get their patients hooked. They simply want their patients to get better and the wait time to be seen by a pain specialist can be weeks long. A chronic pain patient who no longer needs pills or experiences pain is the best marketing a doctor could ask for. Most doctors were trying to do the right thing based on what they knew about opioids at the time and what insurers would cover.

The antidotes listed below are focused on upstream prevention. For those already suffering from opioid use disorders, it's critical that health plans cover the best evidence-based treatments. Today, that means medication-assisted therapy, although the field of study is evolving, so it is critical that plans reflect the latest developments.

Table 2: Opioid Crisis Drivers and Antidotes

Opioid crisis driver	Background	Proven employer antidotes
Undertreated pain leading to a 5th vital sign and increased prescribing	This concept was initially promoted by the American Pain Society to elevate awareness of pain treatment among health care professionals. The Veteran's Health Administration made pain a 5th vital sign in 1998, followed by their creation of the "Pain as the 5th Vital Sign Toolkit" in 2000. This made pain equal to things like blood pressure – a number to be managed with medications or lifestyle changes. In 2001, the Joint Commission established standards for pain assessment and treatment in response to the national outcry about widespread undertreatment, putting severe pressure on doctors and nurses to prescribe opioids.	Value-based primary care is critical to physicians understanding the issues behind a patient's pain: With musculoskeletal (MSK) related costs accounting for 20% of health care spending, wise employers integrate physical therapy (PT) specialists into primary care, and workplace design and seek out organizations that use PT upfront in triage. *(Case Study: City of Milwaukee)* Appropriate use of drug testing and regular checks of state prescription drug monitoring reports can help identify a substance use disorder and start the process to wellness earlier. *(Case Study: Rosen Hotel & Resorts)*

Table 2: Opioid Crisis Drivers and Antidotes (continued)

Opioid crisis driver	Background	Proven employer antidotes
Pharmaceutical industry sales and marketing blitz	Pharmaceutical companies capitalized on the other drivers listed here. Through major marketing campaigns,[71] they got physicians to prescribe opioid products such as OxyContin and Vicodin in high quantities – even though the evidence[72] of their efficacy in treating chronic pain is very weak,[73] and the evidence that they cause harm in the long term is very strong.[74] Perhaps no organizations had more ability to flag the growing crisis than pharmacy benefits managers and distributors, as they had the complete view of dramatic increases in opioid volume; instead, they let the crisis explode in severity. In contrast to other countries, U.S. physicians stopped prescribing slow and low, one byproduct of which is huge amounts of opioids readily available in medicine cabinets for people suffering any level of pain – and for teenagers to abuse. Direct-to-consumer advertising also significantly increased patient requests for opioid prescriptions.[75]	Let's face it, sales and marketing works. Value-based primary care organizations ensure clinicians receive education on, and have in place, viable, quantifiable treatment options that maximize value and come from unbiased sources – and have time to explain to patients how nonopioid treatment options are more effective. *(Case Study: Langdale Industries)*

Table 2: Opioid Crisis Drivers and Antidotes (continued)

Opioid crisis driver	Background	Proven employer antidotes
Opioids used for noncancer chronic pain (e.g., back pain)	Eighty percent of people will have lower back pain in their lifetime, making it one of the most common reasons for missing work.[76] Stress or inappropriate posture, a sedentary lifestyle, and poor workplace ergonomics can all lead to back, neck, and other kinds of MSK pain. The American Academy of Neurology (AAN) told its members that the risks of opioids in the treatment of noncancer chronic pain patients far outweighed the benefits, yet the practice is widespread. The AAN observed that if physicians stopped using the drugs to treat conditions such as fibromyalgia, back pain, and headache, long-term exposure to opioids could decline by as much as 50%.	Progressive benefits programs weave non-opioid options into both clinical and nonclinical settings. One example is PT for back pain. Another is Rosen Hotel's incorporating movement training and ergonomic adjustments into the workplace. A well-informed health plan document should include policies spelling out certain steps to be taken before and after administration of opioids, placing a time limit on how long an employee can be authorized to take the medication. *(Case Study: Rosen Hotel & Resorts)*

Table 2: Opioid Crisis Drivers and Antidotes (continued)

Opioid crisis driver	Background	Proven employer antidotes
Economic distress	Drug, alcohol, and suicide mortality rates are higher in counties with more economic distress and a larger working class. Many counties with high mortality rates have also seen significant manufacturing employment losses over the past several decades.[77] For every 1% rise in unemployment, there's a 4% rise in addiction and a 7% increase in emergency department visits.[78] Remember, health care costs can consume as much as 50% of the total compensation package for people making less than $15 per hour,[79] suppressing wages and holding back job growth.	The case study about Tulsa-based Enovation Controls shows how a manufacturer with a blue-collar workforce designed benefits that make smart decisions free (e.g., eliminating copays and deductibles when using high-value surgical hospitals) and bad decisions expensive (e.g., going to low-quality providers who have higher complication rates, poor outcomes, and overtreatment). With poor plan design, more than half the workforce is one minor medical issue away from financial ruin. Wise plan design eliminates cost-sharing for smart health care decisions. Increasingly, employers such as Palmer Johnson Power Systems put more money in employees' pockets by educating and engaging them in wise health care decisions. *(Case Study: Enovation Controls)*

Table 2: Opioid Crisis Drivers and Antidotes (continued)

Opioid crisis driver	Background	Proven employer antidotes
Declining reimbursement that increases physician prescribing of opioids	Reimbursement for physicians in private practice continues to decline, despite an escalation of both operating costs and administrative burden. As patient volume increases to make up for lower payment, the average amount of time a provider can spend with the patient decreases, boosting the probability of the provider writing a prescription.[80] The pressures to increase volume make it incredibly challenging for most providers, who typically are not well versed in addiction medicine, to identify and effectively manage patients with chronic pain and potentially undiagnosed substance abuse.	In a value-based primary care model, patients have the proper amount of time with their doctor. An increase in patient interaction time shuts down some of the on-ramps to opioids, whether it's inappropriate opioid prescribing or unnecessary and excessive surgeries that are typically followed by opioid prescriptions.

Table 2: Opioid Crisis Drivers and Antidotes (continued)

Opioid crisis driver	Background	Proven employer antidotes
Insurers' refusal to cover validated treatments	Insurance companies' refusal to cover scientifically validated approaches for pain management such as PT, cognitive behavior therapy, psychological support, or interventional pain procedures also contributed to this crisis. Mental health parity legislation forced insurers' hands when it took effect in 2010, but PT and workplace redesign continue to be marginalized despite their proven effects. Even when a physician appeals to an insurance company to approve treatments that may help the patient, several months or even years can go by, especially in workers' compensation cases.[81] By then, the patient may be on escalating doses of opioids just to function as a result of increased tolerance. This results in more anxiety and depression and can often lead to financial devastation from loss of employment.	Health Rosetta-type plans pay for evidence-based services (e.g., cognitive behavioral therapy, PT, behavioral health services) delivered via telehealth, value-based primary care, etc.

Table 2: Opioid Crisis Drivers and Antidotes (continued)

Opioid crisis driver	Background	Proven employer antidotes
Health-related state/local budget challenges that weaken community resilience	Governments can only raise taxes so much. We've seen how out-of-control health care costs have eaten away at the very items that make a community more resistant to public health challenges; every budget item that has been cut could help stem the opioid crisis. One example is mental health funding, a particularly powerful antidote to the opioid crisis. At the local level, funding shortfalls are exacerbated as tax-exempt health systems are often among the largest property owners yet pay no taxes. And still America's perverse health care incentives reinforce the misconception that building hospitals is a long-term economic driver.	Examples abound in our case studies. On the East Coast, the Pittsburgh Schools' case study shows how steering school district employees and dependents away from low-value (if high reputation) medical centers that squander dollars can translate into better teacher pay and smaller class sizes. The city of Milwaukee has avoided many budget struggles afflicting other large Midwestern cities by controlling health care costs. On the West Coast, the city of Kirkland (WA) has also found that the best way to slash health care costs is to improve benefits.[82] While many communities are pulling back on investments that drive health outcomes (e.g., walkability, safety, parks, clean air/water), Kirkland is able to maintain or increase these investments in community well-being. *(Case Studies: Pittsburgh Schools; City of Milwaukee)*

Table 2: Opioid Crisis Drivers and Antidotes (continued)

Opioid crisis driver	Background	Proven employer antidotes
Mental disorders treated with opioids	According to a recent study, more than half of all opioid prescriptions in the United States annually go to adults with a mental illness who represent just 16% of the U.S. population.[83] It's important to note that depression and anxiety worsen pain and vice versa. Healthy and effective stress and life-coping skills, available through a value-based primary care model, can decrease the impact of this pain.	Evidence-based benefits plans ensure behavioral health is woven into primary care and isn't an afterthought. A critical success factor is removing access barriers to mental health professionals. Where there is sufficient employee concentration, behavioral health services should exist inside clinics. In other settings, it's more practical to have the mental health specialist connected remotely, an approach that also overcomes the disparity in different locations' access to mental health professionals. Behavioral health issues are particularly shortchanged in the rushed, "drive-by" appointments that are all too common in volume-driven primary care. Since mental health issues underlie so many exacerbations of chronic diseases, it is part of the "magic" of a primary care setting that there is time to pick up on issues that may keep someone from complying with a care plan.

Table 2: Opioid Crisis Drivers and Antidotes (continued)

Opioid crisis driver	Background	Proven employer antidotes
Patient satisfaction scores influence on hospital income	Results from HCAHPS and Press Ganey patient satisfaction surveys, which directly impact hospital income further amped up the pressure. Administrators harangued nurses and doctors to make patients happy by giving them opioids. Data from approximately 52,000 adults was assessed from 2000 to 2007 via the Medical Expenditure Panel Survey; a 26% increase in mortality rates was observed among those who were most satisfied.[84] CMS announced it would remove pain management from its determination of hospital payments beginning in 2018, but that didn't undo the damage that has been done.	Evidence is mixed on whether patient satisfaction correlates with improved outcomes or with greater inpatient use, higher overall health care and prescription drug expenditures, and increased mortality.[85] Wise employers contract with health care organizations focused on other metrics – for example, the Net Promoter Score (NPS), a measure of customer likelihood to recommend a product or service and more likely aligned with holistic approaches focused on keeping people well. While NPS scoring alone won't solve the problem, it's frequently an indicator of an organization that puts the individual, rather than revenue optimization, at the center of their design.

Table 2: Opioid Crisis Drivers and Antidotes (continued)

Opioid crisis driver	Background	Proven employer antidotes
Patients looking for a quick fix	An unfortunate part of American culture is seeking quick fixes. Patients want a pill for instant pain relief and advertising has conditioned them to expect one. This tendency is exacerbated by doctors looking for a quick fix during their short appointments with patients. The reality is that most patients hear more from pharmaceutical companies (16-18 hours of pharma ads per year[86]) than from their doctor (typically under two hours per year). With this "instant-fix" conditioning from players across the health care system, many patients aren't willing to invest time in cognitive behavioral therapy, mindful meditation, or a regular program of PT/exercise. At the same time, we've forgotten that some pain is a good indicator of a problem to solve and shouldn't be instantly numbed.	Value-based primary care organizations recognize that pain rarely has quick fixes; there is usually some issue beneath the pain – stress, ergonomics, lifestyle – and doctors need sufficient time with patients to uncover it. Volume-centric, fee-for-service primary care exacerbates the pressure on doctors to deliver a quick fix. Employers such as IBM realize that investing in proper primary care that weaves in PT and mental health not only lowers costs, it also contributes to a high-performance workforce.

Table 2: Opioid Crisis Drivers and Antidotes (continued)

Opioid crisis driver	Background	Proven employer antidotes
Lack of access to specialists	In many rural areas, availability of PT and mental health treatment can be limited, and pain specialists trained in nonopioid pain management are shockingly rare. Consequently, the only tool in the toolbox has been more pills.	As we will see, sending employees to centers of excellence and using telemedicine are two increasingly common ways savvy companies are overcoming this problem. From both a lack of specialist access and burdensome pricing perspectives, the Langdale case study shows how it can be done – and, in the case of travel, pay for itself many times over – in rural Georgia. *(Case Study: Langdale Industries)*

Table 2: Opioid Crisis Drivers and Antidotes (continued)

Opioid crisis driver	Background	Proven employer antidotes
Criminal abuse of the system	In many places, doctors lacking ethics were easier to find than proper pain treatment. Initially, "pill mills" disguised as "pain clinics" gave legitimate pain doctors a bad name. Pharmacy benefits managers and pharmacies were more than willing to go along with the game, making billions in the process. The public and private sector purchasers prescribing databases by dropped the ball on this not having opiate in place to catch the bad actors. As prescription opioid availability tightened up, cheap black tar heroin filled the need for individuals suffering from addiction; people addicted to opioid medications are 40 times more likely to get addicted to heroin.[87]	This is mostly outside the domain of employers; however, effective approaches make employees less vulnerable to pursuing illegal drugs.

It's impossible to truly fix something without first understanding what caused it to break. That's why the chart juxtaposes drivers of the opioid crisis with its solutions, a pairing that we will use going forward to discuss more broadly how our current, catastrophic health care system came to be.

Key Takeaways and Things to Think About:

- If industry practices aren't reformed, the opioid crisis will be repeated. Already, the benzos crisis is at the level the opioid crisis was at 10 years ago. For example, the flow of money through the health insurance companies and pharmacy benefits managers is just as influential as drug maker payments to physicians; at least the latter are now transparently reported.
- Media and education are critical to destigmatizing those enslaved by opioid overuse disorders. If we stigmatized people receiving treatment for diabetes or heart disease, they would also avoid getting treatment.
- When primary care is badly undermined, it creates fertile ground for overprescribing drugs such as opioids. When primary care is trapped within volume-centric health systems designed to maximize fee-for-service revenue, it fuels non-evidence-based treatments such as opioids or surgeries for back pain.
- The dominant primary care model prevalent in the U.S. is designed to get you as quickly as possible to costly pro-cedures and tests that favor health care system revenue rather than health outcomes.
- Pharmacy benefits managers (PBMs) design formularies to push brand drugs that cost 100 times more than equally effective generics and over-the-counter drugs, so they can optimize their bottom line.
- Complex medical situations are often misdiagnosed and addressed by health systems with inadequate experience and/or improper safety procedures, with severe health and financial consequences.
- Rebuilding primary care in communities is foundational to solving both the opioid crisis and the larger squander-ing of economic resources by a wasteful health care sys-tem that extracts dollars out of local economies.

CHAPTER 6

SO, HOW DID WE GET HERE?

W hy is health care so broken? Following the money is a good place to start. Our problems started with tax policy in the 1940s. During WWII we had wage controls, but employer-paid benefits didn't count as wages. To attract employees, employers started offering more and more health benefits without paying attention to what these benefits cost. This is our original sin. It could also be our fount of redemption.

Today, the tax break for employer-paid benefits is estimated at over $600 billion, making it the largest tax break in the tax code, the nation's second largest entitlement after Medicare,[88] and the primary wage suppression driver.

Over time, this practice sheltered us from the true cost of the care we buy, creating enormous dysfunction in what care we pay for and how we pay for it. We ended up focusing on a certain type of high-technology, acute medical care – which we financially reward far more than lower-level preventive and chronic care – without regard for the quality of the outcomes or value of the care. Because what difference does it make? Most of us get our care paid for by our employer or a government entity, which are just as ignorant about the true costs as we are. And here's the kicker: Most physicians and hospitals don't even know what it really costs to provide care because no one has held them accountable for such a long time.

This has big consequences. Our system's financial incentives aren't aligned with the outcomes we want, which most of us define as staying healthy in the first place and receiving high-quality care when we need it, while still being able to afford and live a satisfying life. Instead, over the decades, our health care system has made millions of small decisions to increase the quantity of procedures and pills provided, which increases revenue, resulting in hyperinflated costs and, sometimes, devastating consequences such as the opioid crisis.

A Bigger Bite

Middle-class families' spending on health care has increased 25% since 2007. Other basic needs, such as clothing and food, have decreased.

Percent change in middle-income households' spending on basic needs (2007 to 2014)

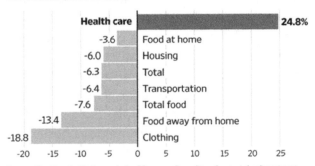

Sources: Brookings Institution analysis of Consumer Expenditure Survey, Labor Department
THE WALL STREET JOURNAL.

Figure 11: The Wall Street Journal, "Burden of Health-Care Costs Moves to the Middle Class."[90]

It's a sad equation: Poor financial incentives + we all want care + decades of small decisions = where we are today. The Kaiser Foundation found that "since Medicare passed, per capita [health care] spending has grown more than 50-fold. This far outstrips per capita spending on all other goods and services by at least 5 times."[89] The trend is only accelerating. Figure 11 is from the *Wall Street Journal* and shows that health care takes 25% more of middle-income household spending than in 2007.

The Annual Benefits Kabuki Dance

Much of this dire situation is due to what benefits expert Craig Lack calls the annual kabuki dance of employers and health plans, which he described to me in a memorable conversation. Lack, CEO of the consulting firm ENERGI and coauthor of *Think and Grow Rich Today*, says employers have been led to believe the best they can hope for is merely a lessbad rate increase – even though there has been little to no increase in the underlying costs of medicine:

"Every year, CFOs ask their human resources (HR) team for a budget increase target. The overburdened and risk-averse nature of HR at most organizations is to preserve the status quo. The insurance companies know this and typically come in with an increase of 11%-14%; the insurance brokers know this and 'negotiate' a less bad increase, staying below the CFO's budget, and there you have it. Check the box, health care can be put to bed. See you next year. That's what passes for health care risk management at far too many organizations."

This system has continued because of two directives CEOs have long given HR: Keep people happy and don't get us sued.

This may have made sense when health care benefits were a small percentage of the company's budget, but decades of hyper-inflating costs have made it the second or third largest expense. Also, it is hard to make the argument that a company is keeping employees happy when health insurance has the lowest customer satisfaction of any industry and high-deductible plans have suddenly become the norm.

I'm regularly asked to speak to benefits consultancies, business coalitions, trade associations, and public-sector organizations about how to tackle this situation. The overriding sentiment I find is that organization executives and benefits leaders have reached their breaking point financially and are no longer willing to accept that every year they're obligated to get less and pay more for health benefits. More than anything else, the recognition that their decisions have contributed to the worsening of the opioid crisis is a wake-up call.

David Contorno is a leading benefits consultant, and one of the reasons he is completely transformed his approach has been the impact he's seen in his client base. In the last year, 22 people on the health plans of his clients died of opioid overdoses. All but two were dependents aged 17-25. There may be nothing more painful than losing a child. These tragedies are part of the reason he's become so passionate about advocating for Direct Primary Care (a model of primary care that removes unnecessary insurance bureaucracy to allow the PCP to spend more time with patients), since undermining primary care via insurance-centric, fee-for-service primary care has been so pervasive and has created fertile ground for overprescribing opioids.

Health Care Costs Are Flat Despite What You Have Heard

I can hear you saying, "But health care prices always go up, don't they?" They do if they go through a PPO or major insurance carrier, but for the most part, negotiated cash or self-pay prices don't, at least not consistently. Sometimes, they modestly increase, but more often, they stay the same – or even go down from year to year.

Note: For the purposes of this book, a "cash price" is what a provider charges an individual who is either paying directly, using a check or credit card, or is covered by an employer or union that pays immediately under a direct contract that bypasses the insurance claims processing process.

We know this thanks to research conducted by journalists at ClearHealthCosts.[91] They surveyed care providers about their cash or self-pay prices for five years and in that time amassed data from 13 metro areas. They found that while some did regularly raise their rates, the ones that did were usually already expensive providers, and for the most part, costs stayed flat across the board.

Just consider what they found in looking at MRI and ultrasound prices in New York City:

ClearHealthCosts Research:

Lower-back MRI without contrast in New York City

Facility	Code	2011	2012	2013	2017
Advanced Radiology	72148	$1,160	$1,160	$1,093	$0
Queens Radiology / Olympic Open MRI	72148	$400	$450	$450	$0
Neighborhood Radiology	72148	X	$150	$150	$150
Radiology of Westchester	72148	X	X	$450	$450
Middle Village Radiology	72148	$350	$450	$450	$500
New Rochelle Radiology	72148	X	X	$500	$500
Greater Waterbury Imaging Center	72148	X	$185	$185	$375
Housatonic Valley Radiology Assoc.	72148	X	X	$816	$627
East River Medical Imaging	72148	$1,900	$1,900	$1,200	$1,900
Columbus Circle Imaging	72148	X	X	$1,200	$2,600
East Manhattan Diagnostic Imaging	72148	X	X	$1,200	$2,600
Union Square Diagnostic Imaging	72148	$800	$1,800	$1,200	$2,600
Advanced Radiology	72148	$1,064	$556	X	X
Astoria Medical Imaging	72148	$450	$1,200	X	X
Park Avenue Radiologists	72148	$1,000	$0	X	X

They also received information on the range of costs for certain procedures at Sutter Maternity and Surgery Center of Santa Cruz for Peninsula Coastal Region, which you will see are dependent on the patient's insurance:

ClearHealthCosts Research: Knee arthroscopy

CPT Code	Billed, Cash, or Self-Pay Price	Insurance Paid Amt.	Patient Responsibility
29881	$15,233.58	$2,681.36	$350
29881	$19,187.85	$3,795.20	$948.80
29881	$13,452.86	$9,080.77	$1,008.91
29881	$18,142.68	$13,607	$0

ClearHealthCosts Research: Repair initial inguinal hernia (No. 1 and No. 2)

CPT Code	Billed, Cash, or Self-Pay Price	Insurance Paid Amt.	Patient Responsibility
36561	$13,950.29	$2,514.75	$641.52
36561	$15,680.49	$8,467.46	$940.83
36561	$15,948.16	$11,961.10	$0

CPT Code	Billed, Cash, or Self-Pay Price	Insurance Paid Amt.	Patient Responsibility
49505	$22,183.85	$3,008.58	$767.50
49505	$17,011.54	$4,576	$1,144
49505	$18,193.78	$12,280.80	$1,364.53

ClearHealthCosts Research:
Carpal tunnel surgery

CPT Code	Billed, Cash, or Self-Pay Price	Insurance Paid Amt.	Patient Responsibility
64721	$9,694.24	$1,953.47	$0
64721	$11,106.59	$3,174.30	$452.70
64721	$11,721.45	$3,501	$0
64721	$10,097.93	$7,079.25	$494.20

ClearHealthCosts Research: Cataract surgery with intraocular lens (IOL)

CPT Code	Billed, Cash, or Self-Pay Price	Insurance Paid Amt.	Patient Responsibility
66984	$10,456.39	$2,473.63	$0
66984	$12,831.26	$2,473.63	$0
66984	$10,878.50	$2,473.63	$0
66984	$10,606.54	$4,328	$100
66984	$11,503.16	$8,024.07	$603.30

If you're not surprised and shocked yet, get ready: insured individuals who ask for cash prices pay less than other insured individuals. ClearHealthCosts found that San Francisco's Castro Valley Open MRI charges $475 cash for a lower-back MRI, but when one insured person went to get the same MRI at a different provider, and asked for the cash price, they paid $580 instead of $1,850. By comparison, another insured person went to get the same MRI from yet another provider, and what they paid was vastly different: The total bill was $5,667, their insurer paid $2,367, and they were left to pay $1,114.54. They paid all that when they could have gotten the same MRI for a fraction of the cost from a different provider.

It's enough to make your head spin.

However, the good news is that there are providers out there that are transparent with their prices, like Keith Smith, MD, from the Surgery Center of Oklahoma. When he spoke to ClearHealth-Costs, it had been nine years since he started publicizing his cash prices. He told them:

"I've only changed them four times. And in every case, I lowered them. So, I think I could make a compelling case that prices are actually falling."

His prices are falling, but he's still making money. He told ClearHealthCosts, "If we realize some efficiency in our practice that we've not seen before, then our inclination is to pass that savings along to the buyer and make ourselves even more competitive in the market."

He's not the only one either – many providers are starting to follow in his footsteps, pushing us closer to the day when anyone can walk into a facility or physician's office with a price and insist they step up and match it.

What's Happening Behind the Scenes

Why isn't this the norm yet? It boils down to three things. One is escalator clauses, which can be found in provider-insurer contracts and which stipulate that payment rates go up automatically each year.

Then there's the chargemaster, a long list of a hospital or health care provider's prices for various procedures/services. One hospital executive told ClearHealthCosts: "Bob in accounting made that list in the 1960s, and we just raise prices every year. But don't tell anybody – we like them to think it's because our cost of business keeps going up, and because of uncompensated care, and because of the burden of keeping an ER open 24-7, and because health care is just expensive."

There are also a lot of people looking to cash in – hospital executive salaries have exploded.

As Smith told ClearHeathCosts, "There are a lot of people in corporate medicine who make a ton of money off the lack of market-competitive pricing. And these people don't want to give that game up."

He also told them it's a myth that insurance companies care about prices. "They really don't. All they care about are charges, because they're in the business of selling discounts. The higher the prices are to start with, the more money they make in dis-counting those prices. So that's part of the problem; a PPO will say that their discount saved an employer tens of thousands of dollars – from which they naturally take their cut."

Criminal Fraud Is Much Bigger Than You Think

Most of us think of fraud in health care as the domain of a few bad doctors, similar to what exists in virtually any human enterprise. In reality, it adds up to a staggering $300 billion annually, roughly 10% of all health care spending.[92] It is also remarkably straightforward to stop, but only if claims administrators – those actually able to stop it – make it happen. Yet, most lack the financial incentives to do so, making only basic after-the-fact attempts that are like trying to stop fraud with a musket in an era of unmanned drones.

More alarming is that significant fraudulent gains may go to foreign actors. The world's cybercrime hotspots are all outside the United States, according to *Time*.[93] *Infoworld*[94] explained why hackers want your health care data: among other reasons, it has a much longer shelf life than other targets like credit cards, which become useless once a consumer gets a new card. Medical and insurance information has value for years. It's bad enough that there is widespread fraud, but the fact that the money is leaving the U.S. economy makes it even more of an economic drain.

Stopping fraud would be like providing the American economy with an annual $300 billion economic stimulus. Over two-plus years, that would be equivalent to the massive stimulus at the beginning of the 2008 financial crisis and COVID-19 pandemic.

Health Insurance Carriers Are Acting Rationally

To understand criminal fraud, you need to understand two key drivers of insurance carrier economics:

1. Anything that drives health care spending upward, even paying fraudulent claims, economically benefits insurance carriers and claims administrators.
2. The ACA's Medical Loss Ratio cap requires that 80%-85% of premium dollars go to care, not marketing and overhead. Because fraud prevention isn't considered care, this reduces economic incentives to invest in it. Technology and other solutions that prevent fraud are just another expense that eats into this government-mandated margin cap.

Even if an employer is self-insured, there is a spillover effect because insurance carriers are generally motivated to invest in technologies and services that fuel revenue increases rather than reduce spending. In other words, there isn't a strong enough motivation to root out waste and fraud.

It's important to note how only-in-health-care dynamics open the door to large-scale fraud in the first place. "Pay and chase programs are like paying a napping guard extra money to chase" a criminal who just cleaned out the bank vault. According to private conversations with industry insiders, insurance companies acting as claims administrators are doing little to stop fraudulent claims. Instead, after allowing fraudulent claims to be paid with your money, they chase after the thieves, receiving 30%-40% of what they recover.

The Data Problem

More fraud creates more upward premium pressure that benefits insurance carriers but takes from everyone else. The root of this is the U.S. health care system's current claims methodology, which is fraught with disconnects and a lack of transparency and control among employers, patients, providers, and insurers. In contrast, the equally large and complex financial industry has been using preventive methodologies for decades, giving consumers both security assurances and control over their credit, resulting in much lower credit card fraud rates – just 0.07% of total volume.[95] This means the cost of health care fraud is 14,285% higher than credit card fraud.

Health care has generally avoided adopting similar prevention measures, erroneously citing a billing and payment system that is too complex for it to work. Instead, employers have resorted to a reactive and largely ineffective approach to recovering money after claims have been paid. This pay and chase method delivers a dismal average return rate of only 2%-4% – enough to say something is being done, but a drop in the bucket compared to the full magnitude of the problem.[96]

When it comes to auditing claims to identify fraud, insurance carriers have historically relied on sampling methodologies to determine whether the claims process is sufficiently secure. Health care claims reviews are done independently on a per-visit basis and are largely a paper-driven process. This allows fraud and waste to fall through the cracks because there is so much disparate data and no standard format for how it is analyzed and processed. Separately, the industry has pushed toward auto-adjudicating claims as quickly as possible, a good thing if not for the lack of correspondingly robust implementation of fraud (and waste and abuse) detection, and prevention technologies and processes.

"The current claims process is predicated on rapid processing of health care transactions with little real emphasis on the legitimacy and accuracy of the claims themselves," states Scott Haas, senior vice president of USI Insurance Services. "The Department of Labor claim processing regulations emphasize the time frame in which claim payers must either pay or deny claims. The regulations assume payers are actually diligent in assessing whether or not the claims require any form of audit or scrutiny."

Such antiquated processes, disparate data, and unintended regulatory consequences create a macro-situation ripe for subjective interpretation of claims and claims data, often making the eventual reconciliation of plan coverage and payment too late. Frequently, this also leads to legitimate claims being denied erroneously, further adding to the frustration of everyone involved in the claims paying process. It's a costly failure for everyone.

Connecting the Data Points

Fraud only becomes visible when you connect all the care participants and events. Here are two real-life examples I've seen:

- A woman undergoing multiple hysterectomies
- A man getting multiple circumcisions from different providers in a single week

Technically, these cases each meet all the basic claims review and adjudication criteria (e.g., all of the fields are filled out and don't have text where numbers should be or vice versa). Therefore, they pass the sufficiency test and the claims are paid. However, it's obvious that both are fraud.

The problems that arise from not connecting the dots can be less obvious than multiple instances of once-in-a-lifetime procedures. One example is a case where four doctors provided the same service to the same patient during the same procedure. When each provider's claim is viewed independently, the claim meets sufficiency criteria and thus passes the paid claims review test. But the total amount they're charging far exceeds the total allowable amount for the contract.

Big data and technologies such as those used for services like Visa Fraud Protection make it possible to identify, predict, and minimize fraud through advanced analytics for detecting fraud and validating claim accuracy and consistency.

Payment integrity technology is available that can analyze disparate claims data at the employer, patient, provider, and insurance carrier levels simultaneously across all health care systems. Such technology-based systems can connect a patient's behavior with the relevant physician behavior. For example, a patient who has had a hysterectomy in the past and suddenly has pregnancy-related claims should be flagged. The financial services industry has used similar behavior patterns both at the retailer and consumer levels to identify purchases that do not fit the consumer's normal behavior since the earliest days of credit cards.

Innovative payment integrity solutions break the reactive pay and chase approach and could nearly eliminate fraud, making it unnecessary for employers to chase after already spent money. These types of solutions will play a critical role in reducing the exorbitant amounts of money lost to fraud and waste in the health care system every year.

Fraud and Abuse Enable the Opioid Crisis

In the area of pharmaceuticals, without immediate intervention to break the pharmaceutical supply chain that travels from manufacturers to fraudulent prescriptions to pharmacy distribution, it is impossible to estimate at this point, the losses the United States will endure in the years ahead.

Governments and large employers that self-insure typically contract with pharmacy benefits managers (PBMs) to manage enrollment of employees and reimbursements for their pharmaceuticals, including opioids. PBMs are typically paid by the transaction or employee; it's not their money, so it's not their risk. They may strive to handle claims quickly and efficiently, but their defenses against fraud and abuse of prescription drugs are antiquated.

The shared responsibilities of the employer or government agency and the PBM create situations in which neither can see the whole picture. Criminals exploit this weakness, leading to a flood of prescription opioids on the street. The American insurance system has allowed this distribution explosion to occur, doing little to nothing to halt its growth.

Of course, willfully fraudulent claims have captured the most attention and are a growing problem. A common example is the individual who fills the same prescription, for the same phantom treatment, on the same day, at five different locations.

Generally, improper prescriptions come from two sources. One comes from fake prescriptions written by doctors for injuries that do not exist. The second is fraud from criminal organizations that use personal identities from breached databases to submit claims.

A Breach of Fiduciary Responsibility

If health care is the immediate cause of the economic depression of middle-class workers, the underlying cause is a breach of fiduciary duty by their employers. While there is a lot of attention paid to the Obamacare exchanges, they only represent about 7% of the population. Understandably, Medicare and Medicaid get a lot of attention, but the fact is that employers collectively pick up the biggest portion of the health care tab and non-retirees overwhelmingly get their health insurance through the workplace. ERISA, which regulates both health and retirement plans, requires employers to act in their employees' interest in providing these benefits. While employers are very good at doing this with retirement plans, they are seriously bad at doing this with health plans.

Could a simple rule clarification trigger a correction of the whole system?

From where I sit, it seems that all the Department of Labor (DOL) needs to do is state that *health benefits dollars are considered the employees' money* – not the employer's. That is, spending on health benefits should be held to the same fiduciary standards as retirement benefits, as the DOL states on their website.[97] That would mean the widespread lack of transparency on fees and conflicts of interest would become a thing of the past.

Sean Schantzen, a former practicing securities attorney who is relatively new to health care, has pointed out that someone in financial services would land in jail or in civil court for breach of fiduciary duty for following what is standard operating procedure in health care. For example, in the class action suit brought by employees against Edison International, the petitioners alleged that Edison breached its fiduciary duties by offering participants in the 401(k)-plan retail-share classes of mutual funds when lower-priced institutional-share classes were available. The employees won a unanimous verdict at the U.S. Supreme Court. By comparison, benefits brokers receive cash bonuses for keeping 90% of their clients in disadvantageous arrangements with specific insurers.

In fairness to the Department of Labor, prior to high-deductible plans, it was easier to argue that health benefits spending was the "employer's money." But today, 51% of the workforce has a deductible of more than $1,000. With cost sharing and high deductibles, employees are typically paying approximately 30% of health benefits costs. So if we're asking them – after taking money out of their paychecks and suppressing their wages to provide them with health benefits – to devote even more of their money to health care, we better make sure it's worth it. Right now, that's not at all the case.

Key Takeaways and Things to Think About:

- The health care system was built over the last 100+ years in response to random events ranging from wars to scientific breakthroughs, creating a tangled jumble of disconnected silos. A fresh reset from the ground up by some employers and governments is showing us the way toward the future.
- Eminence-based medicine (i.e., medicine based on tradition and whom one trained under), often free of evidence, gave way to evidence-enslaved medicine, turning medicine into a transaction. Medicine-as-machine has been punishing to both clinicians and patients alike.
- Despite almost no changes to the underlying costs of health care, there's an annual ritual designed to create the perception that costs have increased. Although it is inaccurate, the misperception is widely believed to be true.

- Prices are flat in the real market – the direct contract and cash-based market – for the vast majority of health care costs.
- Costs haven't changed for most inputs into health care. Prices aren't correlated with underlying costs.
- If your health care costs have increased over the course of the last five years, there is a good chance you need a new advisor.
- Separate the annual benefits process from the benefits advisor decision by as much time as possible.
- Beware of brokers unwilling to align your financial interests with theirs. At the same time, value counts more than fees, so avoid being penny wise and pound foolish.
- Escalator and gag clauses create an opaque market where hospitals and insurance companies have a shared interest in prices going up irrespective of costs.
- Health care fraud is larger than entire industries such as advertising. Technology is available to solve most health care fraud, as has been accomplished in financial services, but key players have disincentives to deploy the technology.
- With guards down, no industry experiences more cyber-crime than health care. Most are using the equivalents of muskets in an era of unmanned drones.
- Lack of modern payment integrity software has been one of the enablers of the opioid crisis.

CHAPTER 7

WHERE DO WE GO NEXT?

I believe the Health Rosetta – an ever-evolving collection of principles and best practices that many like-minded professional colleagues and I have put together is the way forward. It is a blueprint for sustainably reducing costs and improving care, built on real-life successes, not theory. It simplifies the path for civic leaders and benefits advisors to help employers achieve similar results.

Among the former, mayors are particularly well situated to lead their cities out of the opioid crisis. That's because health doesn't start at the hospital or with a pill. Health starts at home, which puts mayors and school superintendents/principals – who, along with other local leaders, are tackling society's toughest challenges today – on the frontlines of the opioid crisis.

Consider how much cities and counties have paid to support things that have in some way contributed to or resulted from the opioid crisis: programs for opioid abuse prevention/treatment, low-performing health plans, overdose first responders, Narcan training, plus court and crime fees. It is no wonder that they have already filed hundreds of lawsuits against drug manufacturers to recover some of it.[98]

Cities are also seeking reimbursement for future costs, including some that historically have not been considered municipal services, such as rehabilitation for those with opioid use disorders and counseling services for their families. They're thinking about the children whose parents are either struggling with addiction or died of an overdose, children who may become the state's responsibility. They're thinking about the emotional impact this may have on emergency personnel and law enforcement officers. They're thinking about how addicted individuals will be unable to contribute to the local economy to the best of their ability, and how deceased individuals will contribute nothing at all.

It may take these lawsuits years to be resolved, so wise civic leaders aren't waiting around. Instead, they are turning the can-do spirit that is the hallmark of cities and towns to upstream preventive strategies. Since the opioid crisis is symptomatic of the larger health care dysfunction, the adage "A crisis is a terrible thing to waste" certainly applies.

Key Strategies for Civic Leaders

Beyond the horrifying human cost of the opioid crisis, the national financial cost is staggering, with the latest estimate being over $500 billion.[99] While that figure is hard to get your arms around, it is easier for local leaders who can easily see the money extracted from their communities each year.

The potential for recapturing that lost economic benefit should be appealing for mayors. Of the $10,000 total per capita spent on health care annually, about $5,000 is being extracted from local economies. That's $500 million in a city of 100,000 people, reflecting fraud and what economists call "rent seeking" behavior (an extraction of value from others without making any contribution to productivity) common in PPO network and PBM pricing, among many other factors. Imagine if those dollars were recycled locally.

We often limit "shop local" thinking to retail and food, but it is just as applicable in health care. One could argue it's even more so, as health care delivery is fundamentally about a local relationship between a clinician and patient. Here are four key strategies for civic leaders to pursue to reverse the damage inflicted by under-performing elements of the health care system.

Use Your Bully Pulpit

Virtually every employer in America, including public-sector entities, has funded the opioid crisis. After all, the vast majority of those enslaved by opioid use disorders are working-age people or their dependents. Unlike past public health crises where a primarily government-led effort has been effective, the opioid crisis can't be solved without employers fundamentally changing their approach to health benefits. Thus, mayors and other civic leaders must enlist the business leaders that employ the bulk of the community.

In many realms, the public sector has been a great second-wave customer after an industry has proven the commercial market viability of a product or service. New and better building practices are an example; private developers were the early adopters of LEED-certified buildings, followed by many cities and states that today require new public-sector buildings to follow LEED standards. Public-sector employers as market accelerators may be the biggest missed opportunity in health policy. A side benefit is that it can take health care policy debates from ideology-based to evidence-based at the local level, where ideological divides often break down.

In the third most-watched TED Talk ever, "How Great Leaders Inspire Action," Simon Sinek recommends that you "start with why," that is, that you start by sharing the higher purpose of organizational change (more on this in the next chapter). It's understandable that both employees and employers are skeptical of benefits changes: first, they have been conditioned for 20 years to accept paying more for less every year; second, they typically won't understand that the best way to slash health care costs is to *improve* benefits. Explaining both the personal *and* broader community benefit is the path to transforming initial resistance to change. Civic leaders should share the Pittsburgh Schools and the Rosen Hotels case studies (at the end of this book) with employers to demonstrate how not squandering health care dollars translates into better benefits and greatly improved opportunities for kids.

Stop Fraud

Fraud is so much more pervasive than most of us (including myself) have guessed. If your community is like others, up to 10% of your health care spending is leaving your community because of fraud.[100] A modest investment in payment integrity technology and claims audits will quickly shed light on the magnitude of your local problem.

Address Substance Abuse

Wise employers realize that the costs of not addressing substance use disorders (SUD) are high. Seventy-five percent of adults with such disorders are in the workforce and the yearly economic impact may be more than $442 billion dollars. Workplaces bear a large portion of those costs through absenteeism, increased health care expenses, and lost productivity. When the substance being abused is pain medication, abusers cost employers more than three times the health care costs of the average worker.[101] According to the National Survey on Drug Use and Health, one of the main drivers of this financial burden is the fact that only 10% of those suffering receive any type of specialized treatment. Many things contribute to this treatment gap, including lack of screening in the health care system, lack of access or ability to pay for care, and fear of shame or discrimination. In fact, a recent study indicated that 24% of those with this disease do not seek treatment because they do not want their friends, family, and co-workers to know about it.[102]

Employers are paying the price for untreated substance abuse in three areas: increased absenteeism/lower productivity, increased job turnover/retraining costs, and increased healthcare utilization. To quantify these costs, the nonprofit Shatterproof, the National Safety Council, and the independent social research organization NORC developed the Substance Use Cost Calculator; they found the costs range from $2,600 per employee in agriculture to more than $13,000 per employee in the communications sector.

Rebuild Primary Care in Your Community

Put simply, the opioid crisis can't be solved without a rebuilt primary care system that gets rid of the fundamentally flawed fee-for-service model. There have been well-intentioned efforts to improve primary care. A Patient-Centered Medical Home (PCMH) is a common approach that has laudable elements. But already overburdened primary care doctors, who are spending an hour or two on bureaucracy for every hour of patient time, have understandably taken a "check the box" approach to PCMH in order to realize the modest bonus payment that rewards compliance with new requirements. The sad fact is that the rise of the PCMH movement paralleled the rising opioid crisis. The point isn't that the PCMH was the cause of the crisis but that putting wings on a car doesn't make it an airplane.

Smart leaders realize that SUDs are a chronic condition, not unlike many other chronic conditions that are best addressed in a proper primary care setting. Primary care physicians (PCPs) can now be board certified in addiction treatment so they can better serve their community's needs. Compared with the financial and emotional ripple effect of an SUDs on families, employers, and communities, the cost to treat and manage the SUD is money well spent.[103]

When unburdened by insurance bureaucracy and volume-based fee-for-service payment models, primary care is the foundation of a properly functioning health care system. Full primary care, a relative rarity in the U.S. today, addresses three key areas:

1. More than 90% of the issues that drive people into the health care system can be fully addressed when a primary care doctor has time to do more than order unnecessary prescriptions, referrals, and tests.

2. It's estimated that 80% of health care spending is a byproduct of lifestyle choices. These issues are almost impossible to address in the less than 30 minutes a typical person spends with their doctor throughout the year in today's typical primary care model. Full primary care consists of a team that includes health coaches, behavioral health, physical therapy, nutrition experts, social workers, and others with the time, empathy, and expertise to reverse common lifestyle-related conditions such as Type II diabetes. Long-term chronic conditions can also lead to mental health issues, which are commonly treated with non-evidence-based opioids and benzodiazepines, leading to further exacerbation of the conditions.

3. PCPs are a vital ally when dealing with medical conditions beyond the scope of a primary care practice. A PCP with enough time is a trusted advisor who can ensure that individuals avoid misdiagnosis and over-treatment in low-value settings. There is no one more trusted by patients than a non-conflicted PCP with the time to fully explain treatment options, and this relationship often heads off unnecessary surgeries and tests.

Value-based primary care organizations, such as Vera Whole Health, guarantee their results and have been certified by the rigorous Validation Institute.[104] In contrast, many health benefits plans use an array of Band-Aids for undermined primary care (e.g., urgent care, retail clinics, silo'ed telehealth, care coordination/management from insurance carriers) that are unnecessary and wasteful when proper primary care is in place. Seattle and Denver are two examples where primary care is being rebuilt brick by brick, to the point that most employers in these two metropolitan areas have access to value-based primary care clinics.

Making Health Local Again

This book focuses on non-legislative strategies because the politics of health care are fraught with pitfalls. As we know, the best way to perpetuate the status quo is to politicize a topic – and nothing is easier to politicize than health care. Having said that, I believe we have an opportunity now where political interests overlap: the right likes local control and the left likes expanding access to care.

Even countries that are perceived to have a nationally controlled health care system have more local control than the United States. Just look at Sweden – the national government sets some overarching principles, but regional county councils (typically representing less than 500,000 people) are responsible for financing and providing health care. This allows local municipalities to take charge of environmental and social welfare issues, things like post-discharge and long-term care; Swedish municipalities recently did this for the elderly and disabled.

Just as it took a while for the built infrastructure to be transformed by LEED, a steady stream of grassroots innovation that proves itself before being replicated is the way we will transform health care in the United States. The following are efforts to make health local again, drawing on promising health care innovations:

- Localized captive insurance plans: Many companies under 50-100 employees aren't comfortable being self-insured, thus losing the freedom to design a smart benefits plan. Localized captive insurance plans allow multiple organizations to pool together to form their own insurance entity. Mayors are encouraging this development in an effort to gain more control and keep money in their communities. Others are supporting legislation allowing for portable benefits untethered to one's job – a particularly acute need for the millions who are freelancers, gig economy workers, temporary workers, and contractors.

- Due to the agreement struck between unions and the Governor Christie administration, New Jersey is on a path to have the largest statewide coverage of value-based primary care. After the pilot phase, it will allow locally owned and controlled primary care clinics to tap into state funds to serve local communities.

- A little-known element of the recent tax legislation is a provision called the Investment in Opportunity Act, which allows the estimated $2 trillion in capital gains sitting on the sidelines to be invested in distressed communities representing over 50 million Americans by deferring capital gains taxes. It's early in the process, but some groups are coming together to invest in things like local grocery stores in underserved areas and community-owned clinics. A good analogy for this is how the Green Bay Packers are community-owned, yet also benefit from an affiliated national entity (the NFL).

- The Accountable Communities of Health (ACH) is a program from the Centers for Medicare & Medicaid Services (CMS) that allows regional groups, analogous to Sweden's county councils, to keep savings in their region when they achieve specific goals, such as reducing hospitalizations. In the status quo model, if a county hospital can reduce Medicaid hospitalizations, the financial reward stays at the state capital. With ACHs, saved money can be reinvested into other health-supporting initiatives such as community centers, public safety, walkability, etc. – all at the discretion of the local organization managing the ACH.

- There are recent ongoing efforts to create federal legislation establishing Community Shared Savings Accounts in Medicaid. Drafts of this legislation propose establishing federal grants for states to provide data to communities so they can identify their top 20 Medicaid cost areas. Communities could choose to implement targeted programs to improve the health of the Medicaid beneficiaries that have simultaneously proven to reduce costs in their top areas.

Once communities proved that their efforts resulted in cost savings, a large percentage of those savings would be allocated to the community shared savings account, to be overseen by a local board, and used for initiatives that improve the community's health status.

- Hospital districts have been a fixture for decades, especially in rural areas. Historically, they have been just as dependent as other health care entities on the perverse incentives of fee-for-service payment models. In places such as Pennsylvania, All-payer Global Budgets[105] are emerging that remove the incentive to fill hospital beds to stay financially afloat. A 50% reduction in hospitalizations frees resources to invest in other health outcome drivers, such as clean water, better food, treatment programs, education, and health-promoting jobs, including community health workers and health coaches.

HEALTH 3.0 VISION AND IMPLICATIONS FOR PROVIDERS & GOVERNMENT

As health benefits get a major overhaul in the employer arena and policymakers determine where publicly paid health care programs will go, we believe it's imperative to take a fresh look at how we've organized our health care system. One area of near-universal agreement is that we should expect far more from our health care system, given the smarts, money, and passion poured into it. Simply shifting who pays for care does little to address the underlying dysfunction of what we pay for and how we pay.

A group of forward-looking individuals have developed a vision for the future of health care. Health 3.0 is a common framework to guide the work of everyone from clinical leaders to benefits professionals to technologists to policymakers. Each should ask whether their strategies, technologies, and policies accelerate or hinder the journey to Health 3.0.

How is Health 3.0 different than Health Rosetta? If Health 3.0 is the North Star—where we want to be—Health Rosetta is the roadmap plus travel tips on how to get there.

Health 3.0 encompasses four key dimensions.

1. Health services (i.e., care delivery and self-care)

What is the optimal way to organize health services, so they build on the strengths of each piece of the health puzzle, rather than operating as an unmatched set of pieces as they do today? Innovative new care delivery models create a bright future that some are already experiencing, in which every member of the care team is operating at the top of his or her license and is highly satisfied with his or her role—a stark contrast to Health Care 2.0, where only 27% of a doctor's day is spent on clinical facetime with patients.

2. Health care purchasing

Underlying virtually every dysfunction in health care are perverse economic incentives. Remember, various industry players are acting perfectly rationally when they do things that are counterproductive to a system that delivers value to every party. The Health Rosetta and Health 3.0 provide a high-level blueprint for how to purchase health and wellness services wisely. We've seen how a workforce can achieve what one health care innovator has described as "twice the health care at half the cost and ten times the delight."

3. Enabling technology

Contrary to common thinking that technology alone can be a positive force for change, technology only turbocharges a highly functional organizational process when the proper organization structure, economic incentives, and processes are in place. Unfortunately, today's health care breaks the first rules I learned as a new consultant fresh out of school— don't automate a broken process and don't throw technology on top of it.

4. Enabling government

At the local, state, and federal level, government can play a tremendously beneficial (or detrimental) role in ensuring health care reaches its full potential. There are four main ways that government entities contribute:

1. As an enabler of health (e.g., public health and social determinants of health)
2. As a benefits purchaser, since government entities are large employers who can accelerate acceptance of new, higher-performing Health 3.0 care models
3. As a payer of taxpayer-funded health plans
4. As a lawmaking or regulating entity

The second item, in particular, is frequently overlooked as a powerful tool for testing and refinement of new models of care payment and delivery.

Health 3.0 Builds on Assets, Corrects Failings of Health 1.0 and 2.0

I'll let Dr. Zubin Damania (aka ZDoggMD), the founder of Health 3.0, make the comparison.

Behind us lies a long-lost, nostalgia-tinged world of unfettered physician autonomy, sacred doctor-patient relationships, and a laser-like focus on the art and humanity of medicine. This was the world of my father, an immigrant and primary care physician in rural California. The world of Health care 1.0. While many still pine for these 'good old days' of medicine, we shouldn't forget that those days weren't really all that good. With unfettered autonomy came high costs and spotty quality. Evidence-based medicine didn't exist; it was consensus and intuition. Volume-based fee-for-service payments incentivized doing things to people, instead of for people. And although the relationship was sacred, the doctor often played the role of captain of the ship, with the rest of the health care team and the patients subordinate.

So, in response to these shortcomings we now have Health Care 2.0 — the era of Big Medicine. Large corporate groups buying practices and hospitals, managed care, and Obamacare, randomized controlled trials and evidence-based guidelines, EMRs, PQRS, HCAHPS, MACRA, Press Ganey, Lean, Six-Sigma. It is the era of Medicine as Machine…of Medicine as Assembly Line. And we — clinicians and patients — are the cogs in the machinery. Instead of ceding authority to physicians, we cede authority to government, administrators, and faceless algorithms. We more often treat a computer screen than a patient. And the doc isn't the boss, but neither is the rest of the health care team — nor the patient. We are ALL treated as commodities…raw materials in the factory.

"Taking the best aspects of 1.0 (deep sacred relationships, physician autonomy) and 2.0 (technology, evidence, teams, systems thinking), Health 3.0 restores the human relationship at the heart of healing. It bolsters that relationship with a team that revolves around the patient while supporting each other as fellow caregivers. What emerges is vastly greater than the sum of the parts.

Caregivers and patients have the time and space and support to develop deep relationships. Providers hold patients accountable for their health, while empowered patients hold providers accountable to be their guides and to know them — and treat them — as unique human beings. Our [electronic health records] EHRs bind us and support us, rather than obstruct us. The promise of Big Data is translated to the unique patient in front of us. Our team provides the lift so everything doesn't fall on one set of shoulders anymore but on health coaches, nurses, social workers, lab techs, EVERYONE together. We are evidence-empowered but not evidence-enslaved. We are paid to keep people healthy, not to click boxes while trying to chase an ever-shrinking piece of the health care pie. Our administrators seek to grow the entire pie instead, for the benefit of ALL stakeholders."

You'll notice that insurance does not enter into Health 3.0, which, again, is concerned with what we buy and how we buy it, not with who assumes the financial risk.

A Pyramid of Health

Health care today is a tangled jumble of silos largely organized around medical technologies, not patients. This mess is exacerbated by economic models and information technology that further impair healing. Health care has been unique in that it uses technology as an excuse for costs to go up and productivity to go down. In Health 3.0, a properly organized health ecosystem can benefit from technology rather than helping fuel hyperinflation for all of us while decreasing productivity and job satisfaction for clinicians.

A group of us are trying to develop a structural model for an ecosystem that looks at health care as an asset rather than simply an expense or a revenue stream to be maximized.

One of our key design points is that the ecosystem should be antifragile, a quality described by Nassim Nicholas Taleb in his book *Antifragile: Things That Gain from Disorder*. For those unfamiliar with Nassim Taleb's work, he introduces the book as follows:

"Some things benefit from shocks; they thrive and grow when exposed to volatility, randomness, disorder, and stressors and love adventure, risk, and uncertainty. Yet, in spite of the ubiquity of the phenomenon, there is no word for the exact opposite of fragile. Let us call it antifragile. Antifragility is beyond resilience or robustness. The resilient resists shocks and stays the same; the antifragile gets better."

We have used a pyramid, shown below, to represent the developing ecosystem and show how various elements of health and health care interrelate. (Figure 15.) Each layer represents a level of care or self-care, and each has four facets, one for each side of the pyramid:

1. Optimal way to deliver health services
2. Optimal way to pay for care

3. Enabling technology for #1 & #2
4. Enabling government role for #1 & #2

Following a given layer (e.g., value-based primary care 3.0) shows how the four facets apply to that layer.

> Note that self-care is necessary at all levels. However, it starts at the foundation.
>
> The pyramid is a holarchy. This just means it incorporates hierarchies that both transcend and include levels. They work like 3D concentric circles, rather than rungs on a ladder. Imagine looking at the pyramid from the top. You will have concentric boxes, with self-care transcending and including them all.

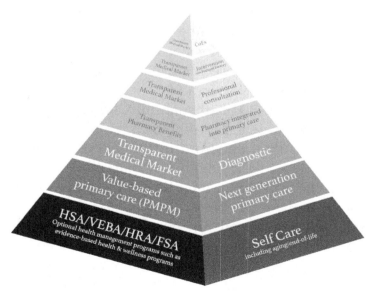

Figure 15: You can also explore an interactive graphic at healthrosetta.org/health[30].

You want to spend as much of your life as possible in self-care at the bottom of the pyramid.* When you have to move to higher layers, you want to move back down ASAP. You read the pyramid from the bottom and at each layer look at the four facets to ensure they are meeting your goals. Thus, you would see that the self-care layer is at the bottom. When you first access the health care system, next generation primary care is where you should start. In countries like Denmark and in the best value-based primary care organizations in the U.S., over 90% of care can be addressed at this level, which includes things like behavioral health, interior work, health coaches, and physical therapy, all enabled by technology like secure messaging, remote monitoring, and other future advances.

If an issue cannot be addressed in primary care, you move up to the diagnostic layer (e.g., lab tests) for deeper insight to rule in/out various issues. Then, if you need a prescription, you'd go to the next layer–pharmacy woven into primary care. Organizations such as ChenMed do this well. If a prescription isn't the answer, you proceed to the next layer for a professional consultation between the PCP and an objective specialist, that is, one who wouldn't be performing any necessary intervention or procedure. If an intervention is needed, you proceed to the next layer–intervention via focused care in a setting with deep experience in that particular intervention.

Jonathan Bush, CEO of athenahealth, told me about his own knee surgery. Even the highest-volume knee surgeons in Boston, he found, do less than one-third of the procedures they could, spending the rest of their time doing marketing for their team. If they spent the majority of their time doing what they do best, they could drop their unit price.

Finally, the unfortunate few who have rare and highly complex conditions would go to a Center of Excellence for their condition (e.g., NIH, Mayo) at the top of the pyramid.

To reiterate, even when at higher levels of the pyramid, the goal is to move back down the pyramid as soon as possible.

This framework reflects the intuitive understanding of the most advanced and successful value-based primary care organizations that two key issues drive costs and quality:

1. Fostering self-care and caregiving by nonprofessional loved ones is essential to optimizing healing and health.
2. Without a seasoned "ship captain" (the primary care physician), rough medical seas cause patients to needlessly suffer from an uncoordinated health care system.

Relatively speaking, I have spent more time with primary care physicians at the base of the pyramid. As I developed this framework further, I was interested in getting specialists' feedback. Specialists, like any group of humans, have many opinions, but I will share the feedback from Dr. Venu Julapalli, who has been widely read due to his writing about the tenets of Health 3.0 and whose comments reflected something of a consensus among the specialists I spoke with.

I am loving what you guys have come up with.

1. *It starts with self-care at the base. That's key. It underscores personal responsibility in health, which has been woefully neglected. At the same time, social determinants of health (SDoH) are right at the base, where they belong. I love the pyramid's government facet, letting it act as the market accelerator, not an overly active market participant without the ability to enable the most effective and efficient system.*
2. *It properly puts value-based primary care right near the base. As a specialist, I don't need to be near the base. I also need to have as few conflicts of interest as possible in my interactions with primary care.*
3. *It properly puts the specialist care in focused settings near the top; this position does not make them the most important, just the most focused. This is what Devi Shetty is executing in India and Cayman Islands—high-volume cardiovascular surgery by experts who love what they do, while dropping unit price ridiculously through streamlined operations and economies of scale.*
4. *It appropriately puts Centers of Excellence at the very top— go there for help with rare diagnoses, but keep it limited. We should also never forget the power of the engaged patient, who destroys the most expert doctors when love for life takes over. See his NY*

Times article as an example, "His Doctors Were Stumped. Then He Took Over."

Overall, I love this pyramid framework. Conceptually, it's honoring much of what I've come to believe on health care, health, and healing. You're distilling what real-life experiences and data have shown works in health care.

Implications for Providers and Government

Major trends are making the care delivery elements of Health 3.0 a once-in-a-career opportunity (or threat). In the U.S. alone, experts expect $1 trillion of annual revenue to shift from one set of health care players to another over the next decade. This is a byproduct of the transition to purchasing health care with accountability baked in. Here are some new realities providers and government entities must prepare to accommodate to thrive in a Health 3.0 world.

Health Care Provider Organizations

1. Convenience and accountability will be essential.

Various new primary care models such as onsite/near-site clinics and direct primary care have significantly expanded their scope of services (e.g., remote monitoring, health coaching). The top performers readily put their fees at risk (e.g., Vera Whole Health, PeakMed, Iora Health). Medicare Advantage programs are taking off like wildfire, with the top performers delivering care far differently than in volume-driven models. If you're a health care provider, this is the future!

We expect Medicare Advantage to continue to grow and Medicaid Advantage to follow closely behind. This trend can't be dismissed as fringe when two early adopter organizations (Care-More and HealthCare Partners) were acquired for over $5 billion and there has been over $1.2 billion invested in next generation primary care models in the past few years. Sadly, we hear of too many organizations trying to foolishly cling to fee-for service and even enacting anti-competitive practices such as threatening doctors in their communities who don't refer to them (e.g., blocking data and patient flows). Our message to you: Don't be scared, be brave. Be among the early organizations that figure out and master how to thrive in the inevitable future.

2. Millennials are moving in.

If you thought boomers were a big deal, millennials dwarf them and are transforming markets. This has already had a devastating impact on a local oligopolistic market (newspapers) similar to health care. In another area of health, big food and big soda have had their worst earnings in decades caused by millennials adopting significantly different purchasing habits than their parents. The status quo in our current legacy health care system is nearly a perfect opposite of what millennials want and value. Organizations that think they're entitled to their patients' kids are in for a rude awakening. For most provider organizations, private employers are their most lucrative revenue stream, and millennials are already the biggest chunk of the workforce and expected to be 75% of the workforce in 10 years. As millennials wake up to the reality that they will be indentured servants to the health care system without change, expect their voices to be heard like never before. Health 3.0 is just what millennials want.

3. Destructive doctor relationships will destroy hospitals' success.

It's not just doctors that feel abused by the Health Care 2.0 system. However, the economic impact of burned-out doctors leaving in droves will stagger today's health care systems. The ZDoggMD "Lose Yourself" anthem highlights the rising revolution of nurses, doctors and clinicians who are saying "enough" and leaving for organizations focused on the Quadruple Aim.

Government Entities

1. Be a smart buyer

It seems every local, state, and federal government is struggling with budget challenges—largely the result of health benefits being the second biggest expense after wages for many of them. As one public entity found, the best way to slash health care costs is to improve benefits (e.g., greatly improved access to value-based primary care). Innovative new health care delivery organizations can serve a broader audience faster if governments are early adopters of higher-performing health benefits for their employees, thus freeing up public funds for the other social determinants of health.

2. Don't rob Peter to pay Paul

Government is in a unique position to improve public health and other social determinants of health—a position that is undermined by hyper-inflating health benefits costs. Social and economic factors drive ~40% of health outcomes, compared with just ~20% for clinical care, yet clinical care consumes far more financial resources (health behaviors and the physical environment are the other 40%). Forward thinking government leaders recognize the opportunity to cultivate what we call Economic Development 3.0, playing the high-performance health ecosystem card and creating enormous value for their constituents. We all intuitively know that health care spending comes at the expense of other household spending. Economic Development 3.0 properly aligns limited public resources to improve social determinants of health and reduce working and middle class wage stagnation.

3. Don't accept in health care what you'd never accept elsewhere.

Imagine if local, state, and federal government contracts for road and highway construction did not insist on smooth connections between road sections. This is exactly what happens in health care: We pay trillions of taxpayer dollars to tax-exempt health care organizations, yet permit them to block implementation of many simple reporting processes and technologies, such as the simple exchange of vital patient information. Collectively, trillions have gone to health care organizations that lack even basic modern connectivity. Nowhere in our society are more lives in jeopardy. It's like military generals who are actively prevented from seeing the full battlefield.

Even worse from a public health perspective is the status quo's limited ability to facilitate two-way communication in crisis situations. We saw this in 2015 with Zika, when health care providers using modern systems could rapidly respond to a threat while those using outdated approaches were left flatfooted. Modern, cloud-based electronic health records and other communication systems can rapidly identify and respond to public health threats, identifying regions and individuals at greatest risk. Yet most organizations use outdated systems that require manual updates. This unnecessarily imperils the most vulnerable in society.

4. First, do no harm.

Sadly, many well-intentioned government efforts have unintended and damaging consequences, too often not understood until it's too late. Government should stop blocking innovations that advance connectedness—stop dictating how technology companies share data and information—and focus instead on rewarding early adopters. Demand that the private sector deliver the right outcome, which is information flowing from all clinical data sources, and then let them get on with it. In short, government officials should adopt a Hippocratic Oath of their own.

I will conclude with a quote highlighting just how badly we need the major overhaul outlined in Health 3.0 . Dr. Otis Brawley, chief medical officer for the American Cancer Society, said, "I have seen enough to conclude that no incident of failure in American medicine should be dismissed as an aberration. Failure is the system."

Simply shifting who pays is just moving deck chairs on the Titanic. Metaphorically, we're all on the same ship.

Key Takeaways and Things to Think About:

- Mayors must use their bully pulpit to convene business leaders in their community to solve the massive opioid crisis. It will be impossible to solve without active engagement by employers, since it is their health benefits that are funding and fueling the over-prescribing of opioids leading to downstream opioid overuse disorders.
- Fraudulent health claims payments drain resources out of local economies, but they also enable opioid diversion. Mayors should lead by example, ensuring that an independent claims audit and payment integrity review is done for city employees.
- Rebuilding primary care in communities is foundational to solving both the opioid crisis and the larger squandering of local economic resources by a wasteful health care system.
- There is no more important role for mayors than ensuring the safety and well-being of their community. Relocalizing health risk management from distant out-of-town health insurance companies to locally rooted and accountable organizations is vital to creating healthy communities.
- Independently administered benefits plans are more work. However, they offer the maximum ability to ensure that plan beneficiaries receive the greatest value and patient safety. Employers that spend 20% less (or even deeper savings) per capita than average, while providing superior benefits, all use independent administrators.
- Leaders should expect and demand the same level of quality, safety, and transparency in health care that they do in all other areas of their organizations.
- Everyone from small manufacturers in rural America to large, urban multinationals can provide better benefits

for the same or less money every year – not unlike every other item in their budgets. There's no need to accept the norm of getting less and paying more.

- The health care system was built over the last 100+ years in response to random events ranging from wars to scientific breakthroughs, creating a tangled jumble of disconnected silos. A fresh reset rebuilding the health care system from the ground up is showing us the way towards the future.
- Eminence-based medicine, often free of evidence, gave way to evidence-enslaved medicine turning medicine into a transaction. Medicine-as-machine has been punishing to both clinicians and patients alike.
- Health 3.0 restores the human relationship at the heart of healing bolstering relationships with a care team that revolves around the patient while supporting each other as fellow caregivers. What emerges is vastly greater than the sum of the parts.
- The most underutilized role of government is as a market accelerator of high-performing health benefits. For the most part, the 22 million public sector workers have health benefits that perpetuate the under-performing status quo health care system.

CHAPTER 8

YOU RUN A HEALTH CARE BUSINESS WHETHER YOU LIKE IT OR NOT

Here's How to Make It Thrive

"GM is a health and benefits company with an auto company attached." – Warren Buffett

GM spends more on health care than steel, just as Starbucks spends more on health care than coffee beans.

For most companies, health care is the second largest expense after payroll. This puts you in the health care business.

So, how's your health care business doing?

When the COO of one large private equity fund's health care benefits purchasing group sits down with the CEO of a newly acquired company, say a manufacturer, that is the first question he asks. Naturally, the CEO will look puzzled. The COO will then show that the company has, for example, 4,200 members enrolled in their health plan and spends the typical $10,000 per year per member for health care. He then rephrases the question: "How's your $42 million health care business?"

That's when the light bulb goes on, said the COO.

A Shift in Mindset

As we have seen, most organizations don't apply the same level of care to their health care spending that they do to other large expenditures. Estimates of fraud, waste, and abuse in health care range from a low of 30% (Institute of Medicine) to over 50% (PwC) but are little known among employers. Note that these are the same companies that often manage other major budget items down to the hundredths of a percent, yet regularly accept 5% to 20% annual health care cost increases. In most cases, they have an overburdened, outgunned HR leader who is overseeing the health care spend with little or no analytic capabilities.

The reality is most companies wouldn't hire their present benefits leader to run a multimillion dollar business unit or product. Then why are they running a multimillion dollar benefits spend?

So, what's different about employers who are winning the battle to slay the health care cost beast? It's all about mindset. It's about waking up to the understanding that improving the value of health benefits is the best way to improve the well-being of their employees while boosting the company's bottom line—and then committing to that path.

In virtually every case, the COO said, employers who have seen the light and taken action see their health care costs flatten or decline a bit while other employers continue to face ever-increasing care costs. Soon they're spending 20% less on health benefits per capita. Eventually, the most successful are spending 40%-55% less. Plus, the financial and other advantages of waking up compound over time. As each year passes, the gap between wide-awake employers and those accepting the status quo grows.

As I've traveled to every corner of the country, I've seen wide-awake employers—large and small, rural and urban, public and private sector—who refuse to buy into what I believe has become the biggest lie in health care: that health care costs can't be controlled.

However, it's not just about costs. We've long heard leaders state that employees are their most important asset. These wide-awake employers, from IBM to a small poultry processor in rural

Wisconsin, have shifted their benefits mindset to match. Instead of looking at health benefits as a soft HR benefit, they now see them as investments in health and well-being that are strategic inputs to their supply chain and P&L. They manage health benefits programs accordingly.

Fair Trade for Health Care

In choosing care provider partners, wide-awake employers understand that the well-being of caregivers has a direct impact on the care of their employees. It's enlightened self-interest to make sure that physicians and other clinical staff are not abused by administrators, working conditions, compensation models, unbridled profit incentives, and other challenges that are, sadly, very common. If the people running the show exhibit disdain for their own staff, how do you think they'll treat yours?

If you've ever bought Fair Trade coffee, you've probably done so in a deliberate effort to say no to products produced by child or slave labor, or whose owners run roughshod over the environment. I'm proposing that you likewise insist that health care organizations exhibit fair and ethical treatment of clinicians and patients before you become one of the latter. Here's what Fair Trade for health care should include.

- *Transparent prices.* Upfront pricing should be readily available without having to subscribe to a special service. Hospitals, physicians, and labs should have continued freedom to set their own prices, but predatory pricing, with a different rate for each person, is out of the question.
- *Bundled prices.* Imagine buying a car and getting a bill for the transmission six months later. You'd be livid, yet this sort of thing happens all the time in the health care industry. A transparent price must include the full bundle of services that wrap around it. This is the

norm for the transparent medical markets we discuss later in this book. While not every last area of health care will fit into a bundle, it's broader than you might imagine. For example, the University of Oklahoma's Harold Hamm Diabetes Center has an all-in bundle for diabetes management at different severity levels.

- *A culture of safety.* Given that preventable medical errors are a leading cause of death in America and bring untold misery to millions of patients every year, one of the best ways to identify a safe hospital is to ask nurses; ask if they would want a family member to receive care in their facility and, if so, by which unit-level team. In fact, the Joint Commission (the U.S. accrediting body for hospitals) strongly recommends that hospitals measure safety culture, and most do, but this information is not shared with the public. Leapfrog Group safety scores are a great source for assessing this.

- *Staff treatment:* Physicians and nurses are suffering from record levels of suicide and burnout—before the imperatives of the pandemic forced them to operate at punishing levels. To think this doesn't affect the quality of care they provide is naive. Research shows that patient outcomes are correlated with how a hospital treats its clinical staff.

- *Ethics-based organizations.* There must be a focus on patient-reported outcomes. That is, outcomes like living without pain or playing a sport—not just having a successful surgery, especially if it would have been better to avoid going into the OR in the first place. Virginia Mason Hospital & Medical Center in Seattle, a forward-looking organization, has been candid in admitting that, at one time, 90% of its spinal procedures were of no help.

While some worry about rationing care, the volume-driven reimbursement system has always rationed choices by pushing us towards costly, invasive treatment options.

Top-performing, value-based primary care organizations tell us that patients virtually always choose the least invasive treatment option first—but only if they're told about sound alternatives to expensive and overused treatments and tests. Equipping patients to become active partners in their own care is the sign of an ethical organization. So are ethical business practices, which do not include intimidating doctors into relationships with a local hospital, an unfortunate and common practice.

- *Data liquidity.* Care teams do their best work when they have the most complete view of a patient's health status. Anything less comes with an increased risk of harm. Likewise, your employees should have easy access to their own information in a secure, patient-controlled data repository—including the right to contribute their own data or take it elsewhere.

Two Stories

In the 2000s, IBM made a mindset shift about employee welfare and decided to integrate its health services. According to Paul Gundy, MD, and Martin Sepulveda, MD—the physicians who led these efforts—the company realized they were competing against giants like WiPro and Infosys from India, which have much lower cost structures. IBM would have to tackle the cost side of the equation, but they also saw that they could gain a strategic advantage if they had much higher-performing teams. Accordingly, they put a particular focus on the fitness, productivity, and resilience of their workforce.

Sepulveda described to me their revelation that indiscriminate provision of health care services—absent efforts to help people understand how to use those services—leads to voracious appetites from both patients and providers for services that add little value but add a lot of cost to the individual, company, and society.

It dawned on him that if they were going to develop a world-wide health care strategy, they would have to build on universal values. People everywhere value health, access, receiving health care, and relationships in health care. It was striking to Sepulveda how important the relationship is between the person receiving care and the person delivering the care. What people understand and what they are willing to do is greatly influenced by that interaction. The ideal setting, he saw, is a full-function primary care setting that includes behavioral health and health coaching.

The challenge for a global leader like IBM was to develop a strategy that would work in vastly different environments: in rapid-growth countries with poor infrastructure, in a socialized country like France, and in a private insurance country like the U.S. They decided that, all other things being equal, they would put a third of their health care chips on prevention, a third on primary care, and a third on employee engagement with (and accountability for) their own health and with the health care system. The result is that IBM has built itself a competitive advantage with a lower cost structure and a higher-performing workforce.

On the other end of the spectrum with a very similar success story is Brakebush, a small poultry processor in rural Wisconsin with 1,700 employees, many of whom are at high risk for injuries due to the nature of their job. For Brakebush, the wake-up call was a realization that they were pouring major resources into one of health care's most notorious money pits: musculoskeletal (MSK) procedures based on no scientific evidence, which in most cases provide less value than physical therapy (PT).

They took a multipronged approach to eliminating the waste, including allocating resources to address and mitigate physical risks in their plants, hiring an onsite PT specialist to provide MSK care in a value-based fee model, and creating a new health care coordinator position to help employees navigate the health system. Brakebush now incentivizes employees who do need surgery to use designated centers of excellence for procedures that come with an upfront bundled price and warranty. They also use price transparency tools, a health care concierge, and health coaching. And in 2016, the company opened a health center that provides primary care, personal training, and a gym—at no cost to employees.

Sounds like a big investment, right? And yet Brakebush paid less for health care in 2016 than it did in 2014. It now spends 50% less than average for companies their size on MSK disorders, saving $1 million a year on just this one area.

What to Look For in a Health Plan Administrator

Obviously, you can't ask most HR benefits directors to pull off this kind of culture change. What you need is a sophisticated health administrator, analogous to the person who's administering your 401(k). This is someone whose skills and experience are commensurate with the magnitude of your investment in health benefits and the level of fiduciary responsibility it carries.

You want a person who is both numbers and people savvy, who understands the inner workings of a health plan, and who can bring real solutions to bear in a way that aligns the incentives of all parties. And then you want to give him or her the clout to get the job done with the respect and support of the C-suite. Depending on the size of your organization, this may be an outside advisor. This person must also be empowered with financial and other performance incentives that align with lowering costs and improving outcomes.

In short, you need someone able to run a complex supply chain. Here are some characteristics to look for.

- Outstanding finance skills with a focus on accuracy in forecasting and communicating stories through numbers.
- Keen understanding that many types of cost-shifting to employees add financial stress that negatively impacts employee well-being and productivity.

- Relentless focus on rooting out status quo health care industry practices designed to redistribute wealth and profits from you to them, including disclosure of commissions and fees, such as hidden bonus structures like insurance carrier overrides paid to benefits brokers.
- Ability to understand and carry out ERISA and other fiduciary responsibilities for administering a high-performance health plan.
- Insight into the moral impact and financial objectives of change and genuine concern for employees and their families.
- Good communication skills.
- Strong analytic, statistical, and actuarial skills to evaluate ROI in an industry that plays fast and loose with both promises and numbers.
- Indefatigable learning, seeking proven solutions from any corner of the country/industry and innovative ideas that will disrupt the status quo.
- Intimacy with the current state of affairs relating to health insurance and health care (i.e., not reliant on information spoon-fed by brokers).
- Ability to build consensus among influential peers, typically other employers and ideally those with large numbers of employees. The greatest leverage, by far, is in numbers.

Key Takeaways and Things to Think About:

- Match the talent and resources to the magnitude of the health benefits task.
- Expect and demand the same level of quality, safety, and transparency in health care that you do in all other areas of your organization.
- From small manufacturers in rural America to large, urban multinationals, it's entirely possible to expect better benefits for the same or less money every year – not unlike every other item in your budget. There's no need to accept the norm of getting less and paying more.

CHAPTER 9

STEPS FOR BUSINESS LEADERS LOOKING TO PREVENT LOANS & LAYOFFS

COVID-19 put American business leaders in a tough spot. Shelter-in-place orders and social distancing made the people in charge of making payroll nervously eye their bottom lines and think through difficult decisions involving loans, layoffs, and even permanent closure.

Some businesses were better off than others, and not necessarily because they were deemed essential. As Kaiser Health News reported, Harris Rosen of Rosen Hotels had a leg up on other employers planning for the reopening of their business. Why? "Employers with on-site health clinics are best positioned to test because they likely have access to the supplies and the providers needed to administer them," Mike Thompson, CEO of the National Alliance of Healthcare Purchaser Coalitions, is credited as saying in the article.

More broadly, the best-positioned employers – in "normal" times and even in times of crisis – are those that have more control over their health plan. To demonstrate the magnitude of the opportunity, consider this: A mature, low-margin company, Pacific Steel & Recycling, reduced its spending from over $8 million to under $3.5 million. The company would have had to have sales revenue increase ~25% to have the same bottom-line impact.

> *Note: Employees also saw improvements in their health benefits such as eliminating cost-sharing and having a member champion to help navigate the health care system.*

For public sector entities, modernizing health benefits is the only plausible way to avoid cutting services in times of dramatic tax revenue reductions. Fortunately, countless public entities (towns, counties and school districts) have demonstrated health benefit reductions of 40% or more when they reset/improve their health benefits strategies.

The good news is, all leaders can find similar successes – and by sharing five simple, easy-to-remember steps, benefits advisors can help them figure out how to do so. (The first letter of each action item spells out a word we all know, "LOCAL")

Step 1. Learn How to Be Liberated from the Status Quo

When it becomes necessary to cut costs, for most employers, the last major area to modernize is health benefits — striking, considering health benefits are often their second biggest expense after payroll. As such, this is the area with the biggest room for improvement.

However, benefits advisors should be prepared for business leaders to be hesitant to undertake a health benefits transformation, because they are likely afraid the change may be viewed negatively by members. That is understandable given that most changes in health benefits for the last 20 years have meant paying more for less and less coverage. Plus, change can be scary and there's always some comfort in the status quo.

Nevertheless, it's important for benefits advisors to communicate that business leaders maintaining the status quo could cost them their business (or lead to services/staff cuts if they're a public entity) and may be the riskiest move of all. They know health benefits are expensive, forcing them to often increase employees' cost-sharing to offset the annual 5%-50% increase their benefits broker says is essential. But they might not know just how miserable status quo health plans are. They have lower satisfaction rates than cable companies, and for good reason: 70% of those who filed for bankruptcy due to medical bills — the No. 1 driver of bankruptcies in the U.S. — had "insurance" that failed to insure against financial ruin.

As we have said, while it may seem backwards to business leaders, the best way to slash health care costs is to improve health benefits; that all starts with learning how to be liberated from the status quo.

Usually, liberated employers realize two things:

1. The shift from a renter to owner mentality (switching from a carrier-controlled plan to an independently administered employer-optimized plan) is a logical progression for CEOs/leaders who have long said that employees are their most valuable asset. As stewards of that asset, those spending 20%-55% *less* per capita on outstanding benefits packages, have shown the way for all employers.

2. Wise health plan design isn't complex and has been successfully tackled in case studies we've published from employers as small as seven employees to many thousands. Michael Lewis put it well, "If it wasn't complicated — it wouldn't be allowed to happen. The complexity disguises what's happening. If it's so complicated that you can't understand it — then you can't question it."

In line with item one, liberated employers cut ties with their status quo plan from an old-line insurance carrier. In an employer-optimized plan, the company directly pays for its employees' medical claims. In reality, it was already paying for them before but with middlemen taking exorbitant fees. Did you know that clinicians — doctors, nurses, PTs, etc. — only get $0.27 of every dollar ostensibly spent on healthcare?

And expanding on item two, I know that all this is possible because I've seen it play out with my own two eyes in every corner of the country. In public and private employers both large and small, health plans that follow the Health Rosetta framework really do accomplish what they claim. Highlighting success stories can prove powerful for benefits advisors trying to convince business leaders to carry on with a health benefits transformation.

Step 2. Optimize Health Plan Infrastructure

Once leaders liberate themself from the status quo, they'll probably feel a few things, empowered and exhilarated, but also daunted about what to do next. That's why step 2 is all about picking the right people and tools to help.

As vital as this step is, it can get a bit technical and boring since it concerns the underpinnings of the health plan. However, if business leaders do a good job selecting a properly aligned benefits advisor, they will not have to deal first-hand with many of these "in-the-weeds" issues.

We know that not all benefits professionals are the same. Unfortunately, the model of the industry has been to have benefits brokers paid by carriers, pharmacy benefits managers (PBMs) and others who have a fiduciary duty to their shareholders to have healthcare spending increase — we find as many as 17 undisclosed revenue streams where someone purporting to represent a buyer earns their income from sellers. Obviously, this works directly against business leaders and other health care purchasers.

Leaders who are taking the next step to liberate themselves from the status quo need to make sure they have a benefits professional that is going to work in their best interest. Asking their current benefits broker the following three questions is a good start, as I have previously described to *Entrepreneur*:

1. What kind of commissions and bonuses do you receive from carriers, in total? *Note: Be sure to ask about indirect compensation they or their brokerage firm may receive from carriers or PBMs.*
2. Do you receive more than half of your compensation from one carrier?
3. Can you meet with me now?

Questions one and two help leaders ensure their benefits professional is most incentivized to help them. The third is more a question of strategy, because the longer their broker delays their time to meet, the less time the business leader has to shop elsewhere. It's a common trick that can put business leaders in a tough spot.

Any ethical benefits broker will happily complete this simple compensation disclosure form, attesting where they or their office receives compensation. If an organization's broker is not willing to share this information, nor meet early and often to discuss options, it is time to find someone new.

Even if an organization's broker does have the "right" answers to the above questions, managing an employer-optimized plan that improves outcomes and saves money will take a special kind of advisor with expertise in this space.

Ideally, benefits advisors will know to effectively "spring clean" the underpinning of the health plan. They'll know how to spot the provider and vendor contracts that have "gotcha" clauses, and they'll be familiar with the fact that the most sophisticated and heavily resourced legal departments in the world have laden so-called "standard" agreements with an almost endless litany of value-extraction devices. We have seen wise benefits advisors clean out $1000 per employee per year in savings from carrier-controlled health plans, even without changing any of the core benefits elements – just the way they contract and oversee the health plans.

Savvy benefits advisors should also know a thing or two about stop-loss insurance, which is necessary to protect business leaders from shock claims; sadly, many benefits brokers have scant knowledge and farm out this important decision. In addition, they should be able to point business leaders to a vetted list of better providers and vendors, including the carrier-independent third-party administrators (TPAs) they'll need to process claims and make sure things run smoothly.

Step 3. Carve out PBM

Targeting pharmacy benefits provides additional savings opportunities. The average person in the street probably is not familiar with the term "pharmacy benefit manager" — "PBM" for short — yet the dominant Big 3 PBMs are all Fortune 50 companies. In fact, they are so big, in 2018 they were able to acquire one of the biggest health insurers in the world, (Aetna).

Interestingly, there is not one purely pharmaceutical company in the Fortune 50. How is that so?

That's because PBMs are organizations that liaise as technically non-pharmaceutical middlemen between drug manufacturers and pharmacies. In exchange for placement of their products on pharmacies' formularies, PBMs negotiate rebates and discounts off drug prices with the manufacturers. The problem is, many PBMs practice opaquely, pocketing the rebates they should be passing along to the pharmacies and their consumers. Rebates are just the tip of the iceberg on PBM shenanigans that transfer money from employees' wallets to theirs.

Fortunately, there are high-value PBMs out there, making it possible for business leaders to have transparent pharmacy benefits, and, in turn, low-cost, high-quality health plans.

Once leaders decide to free themselves from the status quo and find the right benefits professionals to help them, it's time to start where the lowest-hanging fruit is and establish transparent pharmacy benefits; since profiteering is so extreme, yet easy to fix, it can have a hugely positive, nondisruptive impact on health plan members.

With transparent pharmacy benefits, business leaders and their benefits advisors work together to access, understand,

and utilize pharmacy claims data. That requires PBM contracts to make clear that the business owns its claims data as the purchaser of services, and that business leaders have the right to use that data to make informed decisions.

The best-informed decisions are made when business leaders pair their own data with unbiased consultants equipped with analytical know-how, pharmacy industry knowledge, and vendor insight to negotiate better PBM contracts. This will ensure they have a clear understanding of the terms and conditions that are often the source of hidden costs — even definitions left in *or* out of a contract can be financially devastating.

This is especially true when it comes to "guarantees." Average Wholesale Price (AWP), with its associated "discount," is the common method for evaluating PBM financial performance (aka "Any Wild-assed Price" or "Ain't What's Paid.") Because it is often confusing and misleading, AWP can reduce leverage in negotiations.

Another issue is distribution channel pricing variability, such as mail order and specialty. Mail order prescriptions could actually be costing you more than the same drug at retail. In contrast, some mail order and specialty pharmacies offer services for "cost plus a management fee," which can be far less expensive than the AWP model. So, when evaluating a PBM's channels, businesses will want to consider carving out mail order and specialty pharmacy services from the PBM contract, and determine whether it makes sense to leave all of the PBM services with one vendor.

Using strategies like these, the state employee health plan for New Jersey has already saved over $2 billion on drug spending. Caterpillar didn't see overall healthcare costs go up for a decade despite only focusing on drug procurement. Pacific Steel's Rx procurement strategy was a big part of their effort to rid themselves of profiteering and resulted in dropping their spending by more than 50%. And many much smaller health plans are seeing similar savings using exclusively high-value PBMs. Our movement's experience has been that pharmacy spending can be cut 20%-30%, resulting in an overall health care spending reduction of 5%-10% depending on how heavily drugs are used in a health plan.

All this is a testament to the fact that knowledge is, indeed, power in a health benefits transformation. What's equally powerful, however, is value-based primary care.

Step 4. Add Value-Based Primary Care

There is no well-functioning health care system in the world not built on proper primary care. The same can be said about health plans.

The difference between "proper" and "improper" primary care is a matter of fee-for-service (FFS) primary care versus value-based primary care (VBPC). The former is sadly the status quo, in which most primary care practices are owned by health systems/private-equity firms and serve as milk-in-the-back-of-the-store to drive patients to high margin services.

In this fee-for-service system, every service and procedure have a charge — and businesses are billed for each regardless of how helpful they are to the beneficiary. As a result of this flawed incentive structure, primary care appointments are usually very short and often drive referrals to unnecessary, high-margin services such as scans and specialists. It also has a tendency to result in an over-reliance on prescriptions.

While Steps 1-3 are changes that can be made invisible to the employee, this step is clearly visible to members — in an incredibly positive way! Did you know that 75% of Americans surveyed didn't have a relationship with a primary care physician? A Walmart vice president shared that surveyed shoppers (each week they see 140 million Americans) who were asked if they had a relationship with a primary care physician, and only 50% said they did. Of the 50% who said they did, only half could name their doctor or said they had seen him or her in the last two years. Outdated health plans have enabled this and systematically decimated primary care over the last two decades.

By comparison, in a value-based system, providers typically

charge a monthly, quarterly, or annual membership fee that covers all or most primary care services including acute and preventive care. The fee is paid out of an individual's own pocket, by a sponsoring organization such as an employer or union, or by a health plan offering commercial or government programs, such as a Medicare Advantage plan.

Most commonly, the practice has been devoted to the particular sponsoring entity (e.g., an onsite or near-site clinic for employers/unions), but models that serve multiple clients are maturing. Direct primary care (DPC), which offers care directly to individuals, plan administrators, and employers in a range of practice models from solo practitioners to national organizations, is one example of that.

Without the overhead that FFS carries, VBPC practices can offer a more proactive care model that delivers a substantially better experience for patients, often in one or more of the following ways:

- More time with their provider
- Same day appointments
- Short or no wait times in the office
- Better technology, e.g., email, texting, video chats, and other digital-based interactions
- 24/7 coverage by a professional with access to their electronic health record
- Far more coordinated care
- Improved provider experience and professional satisfaction, which, in turn, is known to improve the quality of care

From a business standpoint, this model can also lead to significant reductions in downstream costs. The better-quality care from the outset means less follow-up care — and associated spending — is needed later. And when the focus shifts from reactive, episodic care to a continuous care relationship that takes lifestyle factors and chronic illness into consideration, higher-quality, preventive care management will lead to better health outcomes — and potentially less spending — year over year.

When coupled with the other steps, organizations such as the Bennett School District, Pacific Steel, and Rosen Hotels are literally spending half what other employers are spending per capita. For a low-margin business, that can mean the equivalent of a 25% increase in sales revenue. For a budget constrained organization such as a school district, it's the difference between maintaining programs and providing teacher raises versus what's happening in too many school districts — cut programs and cost-shifting to teachers.

I've seen multiple organizations — and even entire communities — transformed by employers prioritizing value-based primary care and using saved dollars for higher and better purposes (see books and website for case studies), none better than Rosen Hotels. My TED talk takes a deeper dive into the details, but in short: Rosen Hotels spends 55% less per capita on health benefits than the average employer, connecting their employees to not only value-based primary care physicians, but physical therapists, behavioral health specialists, health coaches, and other health professionals.

Step 5. Leave Behind Value-Extracting PPO networks

At this point, leaders may be wondering, *"What about all the other clinics and hospitals outside primary care my employees might have to visit? How will I be able to ensure lower-cost, high-quality care in other areas?"*

The answer savvy benefits advisors will be: Do not stick with your old PPO network. In fact, the physicians described in Step 4 are aware of this and are integral in guiding their patients to high-value health care delivery organizations.

Wise health care purchasers evaluate pricing in health care by looking at what is being charged as a percentage of Medicare pricing. Why? Because Medicare uses a rigorous process to develop pricing that considers actual hospital costs (which are often inflated) and market variances. It is common for PPO network pricing to be 3–5 times Medicare rates or, as it is often called, "300% of Medicare" or "500% of Medicare." Yes, you read that right. Despite hospitals being legally bound to report costs to the federal government that Medicare rates cover, they price gouge at many times that rate. While there are some markets where average commercial payer pricing is lower, there are many more where the number is significantly greater — as high as 1,000% of Medicare in some places. In contrast, independently owned medical practices typically are paid between 90%–120% of Medicare rates and are quite profitable.

Note: Rural and critical access hospitals are exempted from these generalizations. They refer to well-heeled hospitals in urban centers and the suburbs.

A common trope by highly profitable hospital chains is to claim they "lose" money on Medicare. Despite health outcomes that are inferior to the rest of the developed world, U.S. hospitals charge far more than the rest of the world on just about everything. Said another way, they are very inefficient operations. At a recent Health Rosetta Summit, one of Fortune's 50 Greatest Leaders, Marilyn Bartlett, reported on the "Follow the money" study she has been doing for RAND. She outlined the myriad other payments hospitals — especially tax-exempt hospitals — receive that cover so-called "underpayment" by Medicare and Medicaid that are often left out of calculations. They also leave out the vast sums many make through a program called the 340B program that allows tax-exempt hospitals to get extremely low pricing from pharmaceutical companies, yet they charge the typical high prices to employers. In other words, the profit shifts from the pharmaceutical company to the hospital.

To add insult to injury, PPO networks charge access fees of $12-$20 per employee per month (PEPM) for what you might call the privilege of wildly overpaying for health care services. The story insurance carriers continue to push on employers is that their employees won't be able to see a doctor or be admitted to a hospital outside the PPO network relationship. This is every bit as ludicrous as it sounds. Care provider organizations are often eager to develop direct payment arrangements that are far better than typical PPO rates.

The business leaders that choose to take care provider organizations up on that offer through reference-based pricing — where they shop around and negotiate for prices for certain procedures/services off of what Medicare pays — will often pay roughly 150% of Medicare rates. Their logic is that the government has arrived at a price that would enable health care organizations to sustain themselves, so hospitals should be willing to take a 50% premium on top of that. Some accept 120% or less— still far better than what the PPO offers.

With some help from Health Rosetta-certified benefits advisor Scott Haas, Pacific Steel did this and cut spending in half. By directly contracting with nearly 5,000 provider organizations, which were more than happy to do direct deals, Pacific Steel went from spending over $8 million to under $3.5 million.

However, if a business leader and their benefits advisor is going to go through all the work of reaching out to the best physicians, specialists and even centers of excellence — they need to make sure employees utilize them. Otherwise, all will be for naught and both the business and their employees could wind up spending significantly more than you must.

Some ways for business leaders to ensure employees visit their specified medical professionals is to offer incentives like waived copays, coinsurance, and deductibles. Another is to offer employees customer service-style concierge services. A concierge service or navigator can direct employees to the highest-value providers. They also give employees easy access to the human and other resources they need, including hassle-free appointment scheduling, medical records transfer, and both web and mobile access.

That's how it should be, and that's how it can be. With some help and guidance from properly aligned benefits advisors, it's never too late for leaders to start over — setting themselves up for success in the long-term and freeing up enough previously squandered dollars to get them through any current or future economic crisis.

Key Takeaways and Things to Think About:

- There are five straightforward steps to improving benefits while lowering health care spending 20%-40% or more.
- Nothing happens until there is a mindset shift. Most people mistakenly believe that solving health care is like trying to solve Middle East peace. They would like that solved to, but it seems hopeless and out of their control. Fortunately, proven approaches to slaying the health care cost beast abound in every corner of the country, in rural and urban settings, in large and small organizations and in public and private sector plans.
- Hardly a health plan exists that does not need a serious case of spring cleaning. Some employers have found $1,000 of savings per employee per year just by getting rid of junk fees, conflicts-of-interests and watching over claims even through outdated health plans. As employers understand the level of shenanigans in their contracts, they become open to where the bigger opportunities lie such as moving to post-PPO health plans. Without cleaning up damaging contractual terms, some strategies such as direct contracting with willing and able local providers are barred.
- Shenanigan-central is the drug portion of your health plan. Countless employers have dropped their Rx spending in half without employees noticing other than if cost-sharing is removed due to wiser drug procurement.
- The first change that is noticeable to employees is adding proper primary care which many have forgotten exists.

Employees are delighted when they can access their doctor 7x24 and via modern methods rather than waiting weeks to get in and then still having to wait for an interminable time in a waiting room (aptly named!). Let's not forget that it is impossible to price gouge or surprise bill a patient for an ER visit that never happened.

- The last step is the one that has the highest reward. However, it is the one that requires thoughtful planning. In the hands of amateurs, leaving behind value-extracting PPO networks can create problems for members such as balance billing. In contrast, a well-planned rollout generates a highly positive response from members. Everyone loves leaving behind the bewildering array of bills, EOBs (that do not really explain anything) and financial stress of astronomically high deductibles. Instead, wise employers have members champions that help guide people to the highest value providers. The only paperwork the member deals with is a thank you survey.

CHAPTER 10

CREATING A COMMUNITY-OWNED, PARENT-APPROVED HEALTH PLAN

The word "local" takes on multiple meanings in this book. In the last chapter, LOCAL was used as an acronym to walk leaders through the steps they need to take to reduce their annual health care spend. In this chapter, the term will be used to explain what should be at the heart of every health plan: the local community.

Understanding COHPs

Unfortunately, as it stands today, many community health care systems are controlled by out-of-town owned health systems and health plans. That can mean that over 50% of so-called "healthcare dollars" are extracted out of local economies. Yet, the health care system only drives less than 20% of health outcomes.

Often, the dollars being extracted out of local economies are dollars that were previously being spent on education, human services, public health, public safety, mental health, and local aid, aka the "social determinants of health" that drive approximately 80+% of health outcomes.

It is quite clear that status quo health plans have it all backwards – taking money away from the things that would actually improve healthcare and wastefully dumping substantial sums into things that only aim to address symptoms of underlying issues. High-performing, "community-owned" health plans (COHP) do the opposite, focusing on the unique needs of the local community and working to address them before they balloon into bigger, more expensive problems.

Leaders who have done the initial work of going through the LOCAL steps described in the last chapter should head in this direction next – for both financial and moral purposes. COHPs eliminate shareholder profits and/or extravagant executive salaries – common in so-called "non-profit" health plans/systems – as the central guiding principles and mission of the healthcare system, and as a result, produce lower costs and improved levels of care. COHPs prioritize the totality of health – not just institutional healthcare – and provide better working conditions and motivation for caregivers.

They do this by having leaders – be they consumer cooperatives, employers, unions, local governments, or any other entity that manages the health plan – shift from a health plan "renter" mindset to a health plan "owner" mindset. As "member-owners," organizations are incentivized to tailor their health plan to meet their unique needs, or in other words, the needs of their beneficiaries.

The best way for member-owners to meet the needs of their beneficiaries is to connect them with a strong, local, and properly resourced primary care team. This team can help beneficiaries organize and interface with other facets of medical care (e.g., specialty care) when it is needed, and mitigate the impacts of the social determinants of health that could be present in their community.

Primary care providers in COHPs need just four things to be successful:

1. A clear area of responsibility
2. Clear service and quality markers to monitor

3. Freedom to innovate in how to address their population's needs e.g., home care, office visit, phone care, virtual visit, etc.
4. Flat monthly payment that is age and sex-adjusted (in industry parlance, "global capitation" like in Medicare Advantage programs).

This stands in stark contrast to traditional health plans, in which the administrative hassle is maintained by insurance payers to justify their control, independent of medical necessity. Similarly, the primary success metric of traditional health plans with disinterested and distant shareholders is the profit/volume of healthcare services – not, as it should be, the well-being of its members.

The Impact of COHPs

We are seeing dramatically better value from health plans, like COHPs, that focus on the well-being of its members.

The Southcentral Foundation of Alaska's Nuka System of Care is an excellent example. In it, the health care system is built by and around the local community. Its success is defined by the positive outcomes of its plan members, meaning that the local physicians do everything they can to address social determinants of health and empower patients to lead healthier lives.

As a result of The Southcentral Foundation embracing this community-owned approach, from January 2000 to 2017, they saw a 40% decrease in ER visits, as well as a 36% decrease in hospital stays. They also saw overall health care spending dramatically slow: Between 2004 and 2009, annual per capita spending on hospital services grew by only 7% while primary care spending remained below the national index.

Two other great examples can be found in Pacific Steel & Recycling and Rosen Hotels & Resorts. Through a combination of reference-based pricing and paying attention to the quality of care they were paying for, Pacific Steel & Recycling reduced its healthcare spending by over 50%, savings that translated into working class employees retiring with 7-figure retirement nest eggs due to the company's ESOP. And at Rosen Hotels & Resorts – despite having a significant disease burden in their workforce (e.g., 56% of their pregnancies are categorized as high risk) – there's still money left over to invest in the surrounding community. The result is not only better health, it's minuscule amounts of opioid addiction issues, less crime (a reduction of over 60%), and doubled high school graduation rates.

Securing "Parent-Approval"

Health and wellness, crime, education – these are the kinds of things that parents worry about. And seeing as they all, indeed, connect, one could make the case that the best health plans are not only the ones that are community-owned, but ones that would be "parent-approved."

Creating a parent-approved health plan means always searching for ways to get more value; to see better health outcomes, as well as more savings that can be used for higher and better purposes. To do that, it helps for leaders and their advisers to keep Health Rosetta's core tenets – HEALTH (for short) – in mind:

- **Health professionals are incredibly compassionate people who are well trained and want to do good.** But just like patients, health professionals want to see and be seen. Just like patients, they want to hear, and be heard. And just like patients, they want to feel, and be felt. In other words, health professionals desire to be unleashed from a system that does not allow them to love their patients to health, freely and fully. This means they do their best work independent of stifling administrators and bureaucracy in an environment that loves and respects their work. Aligned professionals keep their patients out of harm's way including overtreatment or low value care and institutions. When they have time, they can lay out all the care options.

Health plan implications: Health Rosetta actively seeks out and supports independent, empowered medical practices and hospitals. The "magic" of patient-caregiver partnership returns when administration goes away or moves into the background where it belongs. Technology should be at the service of the patient rather than a tool for profiteering.

- **E-Patients are smart but frustrated they cannot be healthier.** [Note: "E-patients" are a large patient movement that defines the "e" as equipped, enabled, empowered, and engaged in their health and health care decisions.] Everyday living presents many obstacles that can be overcome when caregivers are aware of them, which is why individuals need the health system to be fully engaged with them on a regular basis – not just during visits. Achieving full health is always the overarching goal. That is why communication is the most important medical instrument out there. It drives action and builds trusted relationships, and given the tools that are now available, the good news is that communication has never been easier. Individuals and their dedicated, committed caregivers are the greatest untapped sources of information, knowledge, and motivation, and empowering them to work together will optimize care. However, the full benefits of this will only be realized when there is already a strong foundation, that is, when patients can understand the health risks that come along with their health choices.

Health plan implications: Health Rosetta plans and systems are designed so individuals can stay healthy, taking as few drugs and having as few procedures as possible. Maintaining and optimizing health, rather than maximizing profit and revenue, is always the priority. We recognize that many times, the best place for interaction between the clinician and an individual isn't at the clinic but in the comfort of an individual's home via phone, email, and other digital tools, or even in a social setting such as schools, churches, or other community organizations. Plan design must support this, including using Health Rosetta Dividend money for things outside of the traditional health care system. Health plans should enable a health "ownership" versus a "renter" mentality run by "slum lord" absentee owners (i.e., profiteering carriers and health systems).

- **Avoid waste.** Approximately 50% of the $3.5 trillion health care industry is waste. The more health money that's spent upstream and outside the expensive, wasteful, unnecessary, and redundant health care system, the more money is freed up for maintaining and optimizing health by investing in what actually drives 80% of health outcomes – social determinants like housing, education, food scarcity, etc. Previously squandered money will be there to address the truly catastrophic events, whether a serious medical condition or the need to have caregiver help. This concept can also be applied to individual treatment; when it comes to health care, often less is more, and in many cases, no treatment is much better than any treatment.

    Health plan implications: Avoiding waste allows Health Rosetta to make investments in long-term health. Every health plan should include a Health Rosetta Dividend plan with a dashboard comparing actual spending versus company and overall industry trends. Develop a Health P&L, in which profits include proven non-care health investments, increased pay/bonuses, and reduced cost sharing, while losses reflect increased spending on health care.

- **Local health starts at home.** Local health starts at home and moves out in concentric circles, and the closer health investments are made to home, the higher the yield. It makes sense: Communities are best suited to understand and address their own problems, and when health dollars are re-localized, there's sufficient funding to address those items requiring investment in education, mental health, social services, public health, and more.

Health plan implications: Plan design should always optimize care that can be delivered close to or in the home, whether this means supporting local, independent medical practices or providing tools for self-care, family caregivers, and professional home care. Local public entities (towns, counties, school districts) can and must become market accelerators and bully pulpits for re-localization, because health care costs are intimately linked with all of these vital entities.

- **Trust is built through transparency and openness.** Transformation is dramatically accelerated through openness – sharing ideas, and the transparent open flow of information – as transparency quickly builds a sense of trust.

  Health plan implications: We will be open with the Health Rosetta blueprint, sharing results (good and bad) and our business relationships. We will expect and demand full transparency (well beyond pricing) from providers of care and administrative services.

- **Human-centered health plans restore health, hope, and well-being.** Humane health plans are built on humility, integrity, and generosity. Humility is thinking of others, recognizing that caregivers and individuals together deliver the best outcomes. Integrity includes making individuals aware of all options and the accompanying tradeoffs. When individuals are given full and unconflicted information, they typically choose the least invasive option; when they do not, a humane health plan allows them to make that choice with as few constraints as possible (given resource limitations). A person may have diabetes, but they still want to live their best life possible.

  Health plan implications: Whatever the business or clinical challenge, we will seek out what's best, not necessarily what sounds best or what generates the most revenue.

Often, following these tenets will lead advisors to implement these fundamental health plan components:

- Transparent advisor relationships. All direct and indirect revenue sources/benefits that advisors receive are disclosed to their clients.
- Active ERISA plan management. Employers deeply manage budgets in every other area of spending. Why not health benefits? Internal fiduciary oversight is critical.
- Value-based primary care. Properly conceptualized and incentivized primary care is the frontline of defense against downstream costs.
- Individual stewardship. Navigating health care is complex, even for those of us in the industry. Employees need access to trusted, aligned resources.
- Transparent open networks. Cost and quality are often inversely correlated in health care: Focusing on better quality and outcomes is the path to lower costs. This is particularly true when addressing high-cost outlier claims that make up most of the spending.
- Transparent pharmacy benefits. Purchasers need true transparency of data to control decision making.
- Investment in high-value alternatives (e.g., centers of excellence) rather than low-value plan parts (e.g., workplace wellness programs).

Low-value vs. High-value components

Workplace Wellness Programs

One area of widespread spending that typically has little benefit – and no cost savings – is workplace wellness programs. Promotion of wellness programs has been a particularly deft move by health insurance companies to distract from their economic incentive to raise health care costs. For someone not paying attention, it seems plausible that the fattening of America is a primary driver of increased health care spending (it is not). There are numerous other, much bigger cost-inflation drivers, even if the so-called wellness programs were effective (few are).

To start, they are usually sold on mathematically impossible ROIs and undisclosed commission models that enormously benefit brokers. This has caused Al Lewis, former workplace wellness industry proponent turned leading critic, to offer a $3 million reward to anyone who can prove that the industry has reduced employers' medical claims costs enough to cover its $8 billion annual cost. So far, his money is safe.

By way of background, Lewis was a workplace wellness industry insider, called one of the founding fathers of disease management. Now, he is CEO of Quizzify, a provider of employee health literacy programs, and author of several best-selling books on measuring the outcomes of employee health-improvement programs, especially workplace wellness programs. (Check out *Surviving Workplace Wellness and Why Nobody Believes the Numbers*.)

Promoters place workplace wellness programs among the most important advances in medical history, equivalent in impact to vaccines and antibiotics (their words). Detractors call it a "scam." An entire website, www.theysaidwhat.net, is devoted to exposing its many alleged lies and misdeeds.

Obviously, it cannot be both a significant advance and a total scam. It's critical to know which though, because there is a very specific distinction between workplace wellness programs and everything else in this book. Whereas everything else is an unfortunate byproduct of insuring your employees in today's status quo market, these programs are a totally optional undertaking.

Workplace wellness program fees typically cost employers $100 to $150 per employee per year: plus a similar amount in employee incentives to encourage usage; plus lost work time to participate in screening programs and complete health risk assessments; plus, administrative time to ensure compliance with relevant laws and regulations. Add these up and you start to see that the total costs are much more than just vendor fees. All this to generate great employee dissatisfaction, judging by the fact that a 2016 *Slate* article entitled "Workplace Wellness programs are a Sham" generated more shares than any other Slate article on either health care or the workplace that year.

Lewis advocates a much simpler approach to preventive care: regular screenings based on well-established clinical guidelines developed by the U.S. Preventive Services Task Force (USPSTF), an independent, volunteer panel of national experts in prevention and evidence-based medicine. To balance the harms of over-screening, misdiagnosis, and overtreatment against the benefits of early detection, the USPSTF guidelines recommend far fewer blood screenings, far less frequently than most vendors advocate. These guidelines are easily accessible through the Choosing Wisely initiative, a partnership between the American Board of Internal Medicine Foundation and *Consumer Reports* that seeks to advance a national dialogue on avoiding wasteful or unnecessary medical tests, treatments, and procedures.

Centers of Excellence

Connecting employees who need care to the best-possible places is just as important as making efforts to keep them healthy. After all, sometimes potentially expensive surgeries and procedures are necessary no matter how hard you try to prevent them.

Wise leaders and benefits advisors plan for this in much the same way they plan out their primary care foundation; they seek out the hospitals and surgery centers that boast the best results at the lowest total cost. But they don't stop there and for good reason.

Tom Emerick, a consultant on health care benefits administration, founder of Edison Health, and coauthor of *Cracking Health Costs* and *An Illustrated Guide to Personal Health*, compiled 30 years' worth of data from various sources and found the following serious health conditions and their typical misdiagnosis rates:

- New cancer cases – 20%
- Spine surgery – 67%
- Orthopedic surgery – up to 30%
- Bypass surgery – 60%
- Stents – 50% in some parts of the United States
- Solid organ transplants – 40%

If accurate and poorly managed, cases in any of these areas could easily cost employers tens of thousands of dollars. And even if the hospitals they select for their beneficiaries are pretty darn good, looking elsewhere, toward what is called a center of excellence, could make a gigantic difference.

Centers of excellence are medical centers that specialize in certain high-risk and usually high-cost areas like cancer, organ transplants, heart surgery, etc. Care isn't "one-and-done" so to speak but managed from start to finish. As Emerick puts it:

"A center of excellence typically offers the complete continuum of care for a chronic disease or acute condition such as diabetes or breast cancer, from diagnosis to treatment to rehabilitation, at lower costs than less capable providers. These centers are fundamentally focused on patient care more so than on research or education, although they likely do both. They practice medicine using a team-based, data-driven, and accountable model. They perform high volumes of complex surgeries with great outcomes, yet they are more likely to recommend nonsurgical treatment plans whenever appropriate."

Within a center of excellence, a patient will see and frequently interact with a multidisciplinary team of specialists, receiving not only more thorough care but a wide variety of honest, unbiased opinions about different options, surgical and nonsurgical, in large part because bundled payments replace fee-for-service payments.

Leaders interested in engaging with centers of excellence should start by looking at Health City Cayman Islands, Mayo Clinic in Minnesota, Virginia Mason in Washington, Mercy Hospital in Missouri, Intermountain Healthcare in Utah, Kaiser

Permanente in California, Geisinger Health in Pennsylvania, and Baptist Health in Arkansas. However, it is imperative to remember that excellence is not absolute: Centers of excellence should only be used for the procedures and specialties they're best known for, not anything and everything.

Conclusion

Healthcare is not one size fits all. Each individual person has unique health needs, and the only way those unique needs will be met is if leaders design their health plans to be community-owned and parent-approved.

Once that plan is designed, the next step is for leaders to make sure their organization uses it through effective change management. The next chapter breaks that process down into concrete steps.

Key Takeaways and Things to Think About:

- Health starts at home. The best health plans are those that are rooted in the community and that serve the community, mitigating social determinants of health, improving outcomes, and freeing up previously squandered healthcare dollars.
- Investing in local primary care practices/physicians is critical. There is no high-function health care system in the world not built on it, and U.S. primary care must be rebuilt from the ground up.
- Leaders should look at their health plan from a parent perspective, as health, public safety, education, and other issues are inherently linked. By improving one, leaders can improve others.
- Wellness programs are optional, and money is better spent on what truly drives health and well-being, such as value-based primary care.

- There are extraordinary rates of misdiagnosis and over-treatment that put patients in harm's way. The savings from avoiding complications, misdiagnosis, and over-treatment more than pay for the extra cost of travel to world-class centers.
- The highest quality centers have a team-based model that allows for more accurate diagnoses and more appropriate treatment plans.

CHAPTER 11

LEADING CHANGE

Those who have had the most success transforming benefits for their organizations have realized that great plan design alone is not enough. That is, they understand that even improvements require leadership to bring everyone along, whether they are rank and file or senior executives. In this chapter, we outlined 10 steps that ensure success.

Step 1: Help Employers Treat Employees Like Their Most Valuable Asset

Even if they think they do, most employers do not truly act on the phrase "employees are our most valuable asset" because they aren't actually aware of what their employees want most. For example, some CEOs assume they need to offer higher salaries and more vacation days to make workers feel valuable, when employees care more about something that's not quite as glamorous.

What employees often want is better health benefits.[106] And no, giving them that is not as simple as tacking on an expensive and ineffective workplace wellness program.[107]

One irony is that despite being in an organization of fewer than 10 people, my benefits package is better than when I was at Microsoft during their heyday, when I did not pay a dime for anything. Why? Back then, Microsoft did not guide me to high-value, unconflicted primary care; I was left to figure it out on my own. Like most people, I was not aware of how the big health system in town was – and is – a haven for overtreatment[108] that puts people in harm's way. Now I have a primary care doctor who will guide me to a high-value medical center that won't perform unnecessary, inefficient procedures; one example is the well-regarded Virginia Mason Medical Center in Seattle,[109] which realized that 90% of its spinal procedures didn't help and that physical therapy would have been more beneficial–and changed accordingly.

Designing health plans that cover providers like these comes with challenges, but the rewards are immense. It starts with employers switching from a carrier-controlled, fully-insured plan purchased from a mainstream insurance carrier to a self-insured plan[110] where they pay directly for their employees' medical expenses. (The fact is they were already pre-paying for care but also for a boatload of bureaucracy). Being self-insured, however, will not generate maximum value if employers continue to use the same carrier-provided tools that have created some of the lowest Net Promoter Scores[111] – measures of customer satisfaction – in any industry. These status quo approaches have put employees in harm's way medically and financially, and they persist today.[112]

When employers shed old-line approaches and their benefits advisors craft plans centered around value-based primary care – where physicians are paid for positive outcomes as opposed to being paid for every service or test they administer (fee-for-service care) – they can see tremendous improvements in employee satisfaction and a 20% or more reduction in health care costs. Forward-looking employers are reinvesting those previously squandered dollars, what we call the Health Rosetta Dividend, into what truly drives health outcomes.

A STARK IMBALANCE WITH DRAMATIC REPERCUSSIONS

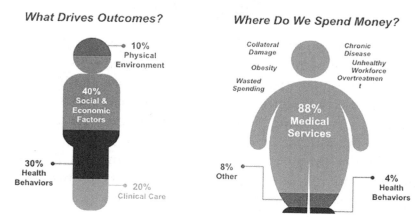

Figure 12: Image Credit: Cascadia Capital LLC[113]

This approach keeps employees happy and healthy; allows employers to invest in the local community or grow their business; and also helps solves a multitude of other public health issues like the opioid crisis.[114] And yet, despite these many benefits, there's still an abundance of employers who haven't made the switch.

I understand that there's comfort in the status quo, even if we know deep down that it is not the best. It is basic human nature to be fearful of the great unknown and not want to take on the work that usually accompanies change. Still, this is not a good enough justification for avoiding it. Change is necessary for any organization to thrive, and we should never settle for something that's "just OK," especially when lives are concerned.

The good news is that I have seen the light at the end of the tunnel. I know that change can happen because I have worked with employers who have chosen the road less traveled and truly demonstrated that their employees are their most valuable asset. (It also does not hurt that their businesses are excelling as a result.)[115] Even better, I am confident other employers can get there too, provided they have the right benefits advisor, take the right approach to leading change, and create a sense of urgency early.

Step 2: Create a Sense of Urgency – Why Change Now?

An unfortunate example of status quo health care was brought to light recently by *LA Times* reporter Noam Levey.[116] Levey helped tell the story of middle-class families who are being crushed by ever-increasing out-of-pocket costs – costs their employers are passing along in a desperate attempt to keep down monthly premiums.

And yet, for every story like this that emerges, there are still millions of people who perceive their current circumstances to be good enough, often because they haven't had a recent medical event and thus haven't experienced how their health plan lets the health care industry extract as much money as possible out of their pockets. They don't want to see changes in their employer-sponsored insurance plans because they've been conditioned to understand that any change will likely make things worse; legacy insurance carriers are good at using FUD tactics[117] to keep their accounts.

The COVID-19 pandemic has also highlighted the failings of and collateral damage from status quo approaches to health plans. As outlined earlier in the book, the pandemic was made worse by a hospital-centric system that devastated the most effective methods of slowing pandemics – strong public health departments and proper primary care. Since most Americans don't have ongoing relationships with a primary care physician anymore, they end up in the hospital where there is already infection and potentially an overburdened facility.

That is why it's crucial for benefits advisors to help employers take employees through the following stages:

Request Suspension of Disbelief

First, employers must ask that individuals suspend their current beliefs about health care finance and delivery as simply not true, backing this up with a data-driven explanation of how health care actually works and its impact on their well-being, and, critically, assuring them that there's already a broadly proven solution – one that will reward their patience and cooperation.

Outline Dysfunction

People will be most moved when they stop thinking of health care as the medium through which their ailments are (hopefully) cured and start viewing it as a poorly run business instead. In effect, it is by far the worst-performing supply chain partner for most organizations. After all, in what other sector would we accept paying more and getting less every year? Learning that their hard-earned, high-deductible dollars feed into a system that's one-third[118] to one-half[119] waste – that adds no value and is often harmful – will get their interest, believe me. Showing them how the current fee-for-service system is rigged against them[120] and is unsustainable in the long-term will light a fire.

Employers should remind workers that the U.S. is the undisputed world leader in medical-bill-driven bankruptcy – the No. 1 cause of bankruptcy for Americans. What is worse, 70% of those people had health insurance. This is because status quo health plans have used a blame-the-victim approach to health plan design.

Soon, employees will start to connect the dots. That time they got a surprise bill in the mail and weren't sure why a visit to an in-network hospital left them with a thousand-dollar balance? How difficult it always seems to be to make a primary care appointment? And how once they get in, tests are done but they are not cured and must go back later? When the inefficiencies and lack of transparency add up, everything will start making sense.

While those wheels are turning, benefits advisors can help employers really drive home their argument by reiterating the fact that they are all paying dearly for this very low-quality, high-cost care. Even worse, the money being spent is money coming out of wages; since 2008, employee family premiums have increased by 55%, two times faster than wages and three times faster than inflation, but doctors and nurses aren't seeing the increase in their own compensation.[121] The median household spends more on hospitals – not health care overall, just hospitals – than on federal taxes. You might call this taxation without representation.

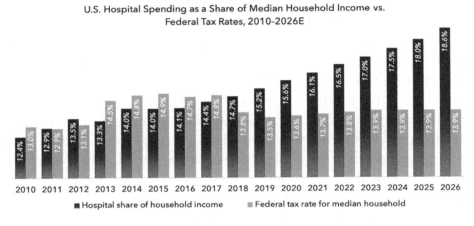

Figure 13: "In 2018, the Average Family Paid More to Hospitals than to the Federal Government in Taxes."[122]

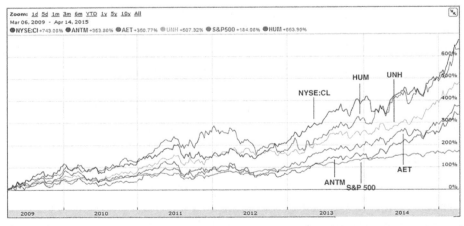

Figure 14: Stock price history for publicly traded health insurance companies and S&P index, March 6, 2009 to April 14, 2015

Where have those hard-earned dollars gone then? The graphic above will give you a clue. That's stock growth that Jeff Bezos would be proud of.

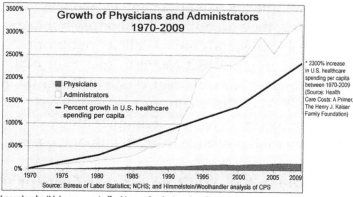

Figure 15: "Senator Sanders: No, Saving Hospitals Actually Isn't a Solution to Our Broken Healthcare System."[123]

Employees need to understand the wealth transfer from the working and middle class to a wildly underperforming health care system. We spend twice what most developed countries spend and have the worst health outcomes, so once again, where has all that money gone? The following two graphics start to explain it.

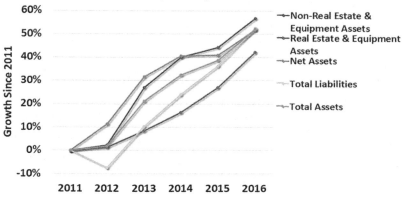

Figure 16: "Senator Sanders: No, Saving Hospitals Actually Isn't a Solution to Our Broken Healthcare System."

Note that the tax-exempt health systems not only charge an arm and a leg, they do not pay local or federal taxes: 7 of the 10 most profitable hospitals are so-called "nonprofits." Often profits are buried in more real estate to fuel their edifice complex, taking even more valuable real estate off local tax rolls. Meanwhile, the CEOs of these tax-exempt health systems are among the most highly compensated, demonstrating a complete disconnect between high pay and strong health outcomes.

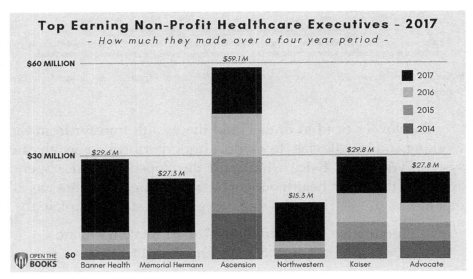

Figure 17: "Top U.S. 'Non-Profit' Hospitals & CEOs Are Racking Up Huge Profits."[124]

The other destination of 20 years' worth of lost wage increases for the working and middle class is in the pharmaceutical arena. Not to let the drug companies off the hook, but do employees know that eight of the Fortune 50 companies primary or most profitable business isn't from making drugs, but administering drug plans (e.g., distributors and PBMs)?

Make It Meaningful

Employees also need to understand the long-term effects of a standard health plan. That explanation starts with a description of what care delivery looks like in the status quo fee-for-service care setting, where providers aren't held accountable for outcomes and where their health system often pushes them to order unnecessary and even harmful tests and procedures. To show them just how devastating this can be when replicated across the entire country, employers should make crystal clear the connection to today's opioid crisis – a self-inflicted wound by a wildly dysfunctional health care system paid for by dollars that should be in the employees' pocketbooks.

Especially if employees have children of their own, this example will really resonate. So many people have been personally touched by the opioid crisis, whether through a family member or friend. And now, history is repeating itself in the form of a dependence on and addiction to benzos like Xanax and Valium, with similarly deadly consequences being funded by your health plan dollars.

No one wants to be viewed as the generation that allowed the creation of another public health disaster, and when they understand that their company's old health plan is a key enabler of the opioid crisis, employees will find it easier to part ways with it. And that's how would-be change-makers get others on board. Knowledge is power and sharing knowledge is all it takes to get employees to realize that health care is expensive and inefficient – but that it does not have to be. Once that registers, benefits advisors and employers will be ready to move forward in their drive for better health benefits.

Step 3: Develop a Vision of Better Benefits

Every organization is unique, which means that the how and why of an employer's vision should be tailored to that organization's culture and circumstances.

However, it is not necessary to reinvent the wheel each time. Here are some visions that have been embraced by forward-looking organizations committed to turning the tide against health benefits that feel like health *detriments* due to mediocre outcomes, poor consumer experience, and the crushing financial burden put on the working and middle class by status quo health plans.

The "Nuts and Bolts" Vision

The most common approach is to focus on the basics:

- Establish a vision for profitability and sustainability. Employers should stress that without change, the company will struggle – and that when the company struggles, so do its employees via reduced benefits, increased cost sharing, and flat wages.
- Focus on the fear of missing out (FOMO). Employers should tell a story, like the one in which a competing organization drives change, gains a market advantage, and puts their company in the hot seat. More and more organizations are realizing the benefit of the Health Rosetta Dividend, where money previously squandered on waste (e.g., overpricing, overtreatment, low-value care) can go to improved take-home pay, better benefits (e.g., paying for a college education), greatly improved retirement benefits, and company competitiveness.
- Focus on how being a smart consumer will help employees. Benefits advisors should help employers leverage tools like bundled surgery payments, affordable/transparent pharmacy benefits, and patient navigation/concierge services – and then incentivize employees to use these services by covering out-of-pocket expenses.
- Create a three-to-five year goal of having better, cheaper coverage. The first-year goal could be to reduce costs by 10% while implementing new, non-carrier programs for employees to use. Many such opportunities for improvement do not take a long time to implement, but it's critical to think in terms of three to five years. This helps filter out the onslaught of short-term oriented, not to mention ineffective solutions that traditional carriers propose.

- Employers should let everyone know that if the organization does nothing, there will be cuts, painting a picture that everyone will want to avoid.

The 11-Star Vision

Another approach comes from LinkedIn founder Reid Hoffman's interview[125] with Airbnb co-founder Brian Chesky about how they overcame conventional thinking with an 11-star system. It's a process in which individuals rate their experience beyond the conventional 5-star system.

Chesky describes the difference:

"A 5-star experience is: You knock on the door, they open the door, they let you in. Great. That's not a big deal. You're not going to tell every friend about it. You might say, 'I used Airbnb. It worked.' So we thought, 'What would a 6-star experience be?'

A 6-star experience: You knock on the door; the host opens and shows you around. On the table would be a welcome gift. It would be a bottle of wine, maybe some candy. You'd open the fridge. There's water. You go to the bathroom, there's toiletries. The whole thing is great. That's a 6-star experience. You'd say, 'Wow, I love this more than a hotel. I'm definitely going to use Airbnb again. It worked. Better than I expected.'"

Maybe employers don't need to go up to 9, 10, or 11, but if they go through the exercise, there will be some sweet spot that's compelling. When the goal is compelling enough, there can be broad-based employee support and "out there" ideas can become feasible.

Even though the organization I co-founded has fewer than 10 employees, we already have a benefits plan better than virtually any employer in the country – large or small. However, we believe we must walk the talk and are striving for more.

For example, we hope all Health Rosetta-type plans can deliver an "11-star" experience in the future that includes these benefits:

- Employer provides health benefits with value-based primary care in a self-funded plan.
- No copays or deductibles for wise decisions.
- All savings go into enhanced pay and profit-sharing.
- Funded college and continuing education for employees and their children.
- 26 weeks of family leave for every seven years of service (can be used for maternity, paternity, family leave/bereavement and sabbatical).
- Free (or discounted) healthy meals provided seven days/week (e.g., the Acme Box).

Knowing that we are striving toward these goals creates a shared vision that guides our efforts. It may take a while to achieve our 11-star vision, but it will help us overcome the inevitable speed bumps along the way.

The Community-Owned Health Plan Vision

Community-minded employers, often referred to as those that adhere to Conscious Capitalism principles,[126] recognize that their community is a key stakeholder in their business and that most health outcomes are determined by what happens in their community – not in hospitals or even the workplace. IBM[127] and Rosen Hotels & Resorts are two exemplary organizations that have acted on this connection. (See case studies.)

THE FUTURE HEALTH ECOSYSTEM WILL FOCUS ON THE TRUE DRIVERS OF OUTCOMES

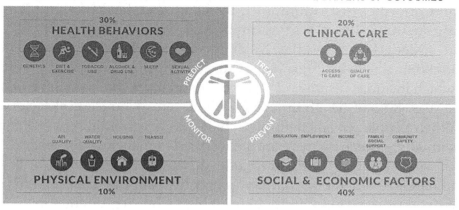

Figure 18: Image Credit: Cascadia Capital, LLC

Not unlike what happened with electrification and tele-communications cooperatives, health plan choices are limited throughout rural America, and the big incumbents either do not serve them at all or serve them very poorly. The good news is that political leaders are eager for solutions and because incumbents do not pay much attention to those markets, innovation can be more unfettered. A great example of this is in Alaska, where the Southcentral Foundation turned a once-failing health care system 90% funded by government programs into a two-time Malcolm Baldrige Award winner owned by the community. They call their model of care the Nuka model.[128] "Nuka" is an Alaska Native word that means "strong, giant structures and living things."

A core tenet of the Nuka model is that individuals formerly known as patients are referred to as "customer-owners" as they have a role in health care's governance and direction. From a clinical vantage point, despite a vast coverage area and significant disease burden, they have seen a 40% reduction in ER visits and a 36% drop in hospital stays while achieving 97% customer-owner satisfaction and 95% employee satisfaction. They're also in the 75th to 90th percentile on many health quality measures. No flash-in-the-pan, this has been consistently achieved for over a decade. The message here: One-size-fits-all approaches from remote, out-of-town headquarters rarely reflect the unique needs and priorities of a community. Instead, when health care dollars are spent locally, all parties can benefit.

Models such as the Nuka model or what's happening in Jönköping, Sweden,[129] are helping us develop our own 11-star vision, which includes health and well-being initiatives that recognize that at least 80% of health outcomes are driven by nonclinical factors. When people see a benefit plan change as a key building block for something much bigger, they are inspired to move further, faster.

Increasingly, companies are driving social change.[130] It's remarkable when one company's benefits plan can catalyze a 62% reduction in crime and a doubling of high school graduation rates.[131] Imagine the impact of several companies in the same community teaming up to solve other challenging, but solvable, problems.

Developing a vision for better health care is a critical step in benefits advisors' and employers' pursuit of change, and fortunately, they have great options. Only with a clear idea of what is ahead will employees see that hard work has a purpose and stay on the path.

Step 4: Secure Grassroots Support

Given the previous three steps, most employees will agree that a major benefits change is critical. Less obvious to employers, though, is how important it is to generate support from the lower levels of the organization. Often, it is people without any traditional, org-chart-based status who can set the tone for how a benefits program is received.

These are some things organization leaders, together with their benefits advisors, should consider when building an alliance for change:

Start Quietly to Build Success

In the words of one benefits consultant, "I prefer to fight my battles as a ninja in the night rather than a soldier on the field."

Providing proper primary care is a great place to start helping employees "see and believe" in the health plan transformation. Even though primary care itself is not a high-cost area, it is the linchpin for success with the other key areas of a plan – transparent open networks, procedures to treat complex medical conditions, and pharmacy benefits.

People who have one trust their primary care physician (PCP), especially if that person is employed by a health system that allows them to practice in the best interests of patients. Trust in PCPs far exceeds trust in health insurance carriers or company leaders.

Build from the "Bottom"

A good place for benefits advisors and employers to start gathering input is in focus groups and wellness committees that include people from all areas of the company – especially some of the complainers, high-health plan utilizers, and people who have been very unhappy with the current health plan. These individuals can also be the beta testers for any new plan.

When such individuals are given access to a value-based, direct primary care physician, it may turn out that lack of adherence to care plans or hypochondria has been part of the problem. Because status quo health plans do not serve these individuals well, they quickly see the great opportunity for improvement. In the beta test, these previously "out of control" patients get the guidance and care they need, and it takes extraordinarily little time to see costs go down along with ER visits and hospitalizations.

An example: One organization had an individual who was having post-bariatric surgery complications that were costing the organization $16,000 every month. By enrolling them with a value-based primary care doctor, the costs (other than the less than $100/month fee for VBPC) immediately dropped to zero. While examples aren't always this dramatic in terms of cost, it is relatively easy to get these types of wins that set the stage for broader rollout success.

If a benefits advisor or employer can show the lowest-paid part of the workforce how to use the plan in a way that saves them and the company money, other excuses about not being able or willing to change seem to diminish. Millennials are especially important to include because their focus on convenience, transparency, and safety – all items the status quo health care system has failed to achieve – often makes them early adopters of new products/ventures.

The initial rollout also sets the stage for a broader rollout where the primary care physician(s) goes onsite during open enrollment. The initial intake should be an hour long and positioned as an executive wellness visit – the same program executives have already received. Having members feel they are getting white-glove treatment goes a long way toward getting broad-based buy-in.

During these initial encounters, the physician(s) should also set up a mobile app that allows members to text them securely and easily. People will be blown away by how accessible their doctor is compared to the past, particularly people who have chronic health problems and think of a doctor visit as the equivalent of going to the principal's office. Fingerwagging doesn't work, as the *New York Times* pointed out recently.[132]

Educate Change Agents.

Once employers have demonstrated to a diverse subset of employees the positive impact of their proposed health plan changes, the next step is to deepen that education. They should communicate the most important information first, including the profits of the hospitals in their market, the hospitals' CEO pay (especially those of tax-exempt organizations who've transferred tax burden onto others in the community), and the value of the real estate owned by the hospital within the community. This can be done by pulling the numbers from county auditor websites in communities where hospitals have a significant presence. Each parcel listing shows taxable value – usually lower than market rate. In some communities, those organizations would be paying more than $20 million per year if they were not tax exempt.

Once they make the connections, employees can begin to see that the choice is between continuing to fuel the massive salaries of tax-exempt executives or finally getting those long-overdue raises.

Next, employers should walk employees through what three to five years down the road will look like if things do not change – the vision to be avoided.

By giving employees – especially lower-level ones that are often overlooked and perhaps most disgruntled by the current health plan – the opportunity to see what positive change will look like, an organization can better position itself to move forward. How, exactly? By using short-term wins to create momentum.

Step 5: Sustain Change and Encourage Progress Using Short-Term Wins

At this point, benefits advisors and employers will already have gotten an alliance of employees on board and be ready to roll out their vision for an improved health benefits transformation. Here, it is important to keep the momentum going, fueling the fire for change and propelling people forward.

The best way to do that is by identifying, sharing, and celebrating short-term wins, which, as Dr. John Kotter points out, should be visible and tangible, unambiguous, and clearly related to the change effort.

Dr. Kotter's work has informed a lot of my thinking in this area. His 8-Step Process for Leading Change[133] is an excellent framework. For example, as it applies here, a short-term win could be either qualitative in the form of an employee success story, or quantitative in the form of black-and-white cost savings.

The following are qualitative examples of short-term wins celebrated after implementing Health Rosetta-type plans:

- More people enrolling in, and taking advantage of, direct primary care (DPC). Despite the concept being foreign to

the average employee, we have seen multiple organizations achieve over 50% enrollment in direct primary care
models that provide an immediate accessibility advantage.

- Praise for care navigators, often nurses. Typically, navigators are not well received when there is not proper primary care available. But when they help families with
guidance on treatment, finding a center of excellence, or
obtaining diabetes supplies in a more affordable and convenient way, word will get around.
- The city of Tyler, Texas has countless qualitative examples
of short-term wins due to a wise onboarding program with
a local DPC organization. Formerly at-risk patients, men
particularly, were astonished to find they had a mobile
app where they could easily reach their DPC doctor. And
starting with small steps, these patients – many already
on multiple medications – were able to turn things around
on issues like blood pressure, diabetes, and back pain.
They were able to get off medications that were costing
them financially and physically, and they now consider
the doctors their friends and allies. (Many of their health
care costs also dropped.)

And here are some quantitative examples of short-term wins:

- Despite budget constraints, one municipality was able to
put $500 into everyone's HRA-VEBA accounts – the pub-
lic-sector equivalent of a health savings account (HSA).
- A private sector employer uncovered significant pharmacy rebates that had not been returned to the plan
sponsor – until now. This turned what would have been
an okay year into a great year for the employer and its
employees.
- An employee who had previously walked into the CEO's
office in tears because she was taking a $40,000/year med-
ication the old plan did not cover was now able to get it
for free under the new plan. Half of her income had been

going towards paying for this medication, exhausting her savings; the new plan was able to navigate the opportunities to source this medication at no cost to the member and at a fraction of the cost for the health plan.

- Many Health Rosetta-type plans remove all copays and deductibles if individuals make wise choices such as calling the concierge line to find high-value care.

Wins like these meet Dr. Kotter's three criteria. They are benefits that employees can see, cannot deny, and can easily relate back to the change effort. They validate the vision, along with everyone's patience and hard work.

When correctly leveraged, they can also be used to drive even greater change: to silence disbelievers; provide feedback to benefits advisors and employers on what's working well, what isn't, and what can be done even better; and keep everyone on track and moving forward.

However, employers cannot just hope for short-term wins to pop up. They must actively look for ways to obtain clear health improvements and reward the people involved with recognition and even money. I know of one organization that rewarded employees for finding billing errors by passing along 20% of the savings. Early on, one employee found a six-figure billing error that they prevented the employer from paying, and it boosted the employee's annual income by over 50% that year. The employer called a company meeting and presented the individual with a giant novelty check, unleashing a small army of people reviewing hospital bills, which are often riddled with errors and duplicate charges.

At the end of the day, short-term wins have a gigantic impact on long-term success.

Step 6: Be on the Lookout for Barriers to Change

Unfortunately, though organizational change will generate moments worth celebrating, it may also throw up some roadblocks along the way. These barriers can be broadly grouped into the following categories: structural, psychological, and cultural.[134]

In the context of a health benefits transformation, here is how each of these might manifest:

Structural Barriers

One potential barrier could be a disagreement between the finance and HR departments over what happens with the savings that are achieved. To prevent this conflict, there should be upfront agreement between employer and employees on how to use what we call the Health Rosetta Dividend: previously squandered dollars that can be used for higher and better purposes. Will that dividend be allocated to profit-sharing or bonuses, R&D, or other enhanced benefits such as paying for education?

Psychological Barriers

Many people have been trained to believe that spending more on care is synonymous with receiving better care, since that is usually the case in other areas of life. If you spend more on a car, you usually get a nicer car. Not so in health care.

If that mentality does not give way before the new health plan, employees may refuse to believe that the benefits change is legitimate, assuming that since their employer is paying less, they are getting less. Employees may enter relationships with the new higher-quality, lower-cost physicians with reluctance, and may even refuse to see them, choosing to stick with their old high-cost, low-quality physicians.

Cultural Barriers

When multiple employees adopt this mindset, it can quickly become a cultural barrier. Attitudes can be contagious, and if a handful of dissenters plant seeds of negativity among their fellow employees, resistance can easily sprout up.

Overcoming a cultural barrier like this is absolutely essential because a value-based health plan only works if everyone does their fair share. If employees do not take advantage of all that the new health plan has to offer, it will not improve outcomes or reduce health care costs.

As you can see, structural, psychological, and cultural barriers often overlap, which also means they can be solved by deploying some of the same strategies. One is to reiterate some of those short-term wins described in Step 5. Step 7 spells out some others.

Step 7: Break Down Change Barriers

People say change is the only constant in life, and barriers almost always come along with it. Barriers, however, can be overcome – assuming you are able to recognize them. Employers need to know how each barrier might manifest in their organization to anticipate and forestall them. Benefits advisors can help on both fronts, specifically by doing the following:

Talking to Both Supporters and Resisters

In Step 4, we saw how resisters can actually work in employers' favor. Here, the same idea applies. Instead of fighting the people that are not for change, benefits advisors should encourage employers to embrace and engage with them.

In fact, employers should communicate with both supporters and resisters early on and often, being consistently truthful, straightforward, and timely. They should use social proof, storytelling, and "what if" scenarios in company-wide emails, intranets, and face-to-face and town hall meetings that allow employees to ask questions and stay informed. They should use a blend of formal and informal communication to ensure that all employees receive the news about the change in some way or another, always referring to their vision and reiterating why change is for the better.

If HR managers are hesitant because they do not want to upset the workforce, they should also be given the opportunity to experience the new benefits program in a beta test. HR managers usually love seeing employees being better supported in new plans via nurse navigators/patient advocates, unlike status quo plans that often leave employees adrift. Once they experience an advocate who is truly on their side, they will quickly abandon their previous resistance.

Thoroughly Engaging Everyone

Talking to employees is important, but just as important is to listen, listen, listen. When transforming their health plan, benefits advisors and employers should engage with employees by asking them probing questions like "Is the new health plan working? What can we do to make it work better? Do you have any questions or concerns?"

Then, benefits advisors and employers need to respond. If feedback is going to be collected, it needs to be read and acted on – perhaps via relevant plan changes – to show employees their ideas and concerns are being heard.

Wise employers will take things a step further by trying to genuinely understand employees' concerns. Instead of only looking at issues on the surface, they should realize that there could be many different reasons for opposition, depending on the person. This information can be especially useful in helping tailor appropriate solutions to work out these problems.

Implementing Change in Several Stages

Change does not happen instantaneously, but it does not and should not have to happen strictly in terms of annual cycles either. Moving too soon or too fast can create resistance; moving too slow and you will fail to build momentum.

Despite their sense of urgency, and along with envisioning change in terms of three to five years, they should set the foundation for change 6-12 months before most employees actually feel that it's happening.

For example, focus groups where employees are asked about the current health plan (What do they like/dislike? What would they like to see?) should be held outside of the normal "benefits season." Then, when the new plan is rolled out, employees can be reminded of the feedback they gave and see how benefits advisors and employers responded to their input. From there, leaders need to develop a roadmap that includes progress checks and course corrections, and opportunities for those confidence-building short-term wins.

Keep Communicating Change

By now, it should be clear just how critical communication is in properly initiating and effectively carrying out change. Benefits advisors and employers must explicitly tell employees what is going on, using the tactics previously laid out. In this way, they can avoid information vacuums and ensure that employees – even the ones who were initially opposed – get on board with the vision, goals, and expectations for what needs to happen and why.

Step 8: Communicate More Than You Think You Need To

George Bernard Shaw once said, "The single biggest problem in communication is the illusion that it has taken place."

It's easy for employers to assume that employees are hanging on their every word – especially when they're making a monumental transition to a higher-quality, lower-cost health plan that benefits them and the organization. But the reality is that a lot can get lost in translation, especially when information is detail-heavy, as it so often is with health care coverage.

Not having a thorough understanding of the health plan, or why a new one is even necessary, can result in employees making high-impact mistakes, ones that could put their own physical and financial well-being on the line. When employees suffer, employers suffer, and this is just one of the reasons why regular communication is critical.

This can be a challenge for HR and benefits advisors. Odds are, they have invested substantial time on the rollout of the new health plan, much of it dealing with technical implementation matters rather than continuous communication. If that is the case, if employees don't know how or why they have to use the new health plan, all that effort could be for naught.

To avoid this, it is critical that benefits advisors and employers revisit their initial message. They should frequently check in with employees to see how things are going. If employees are not able to reiterate why the shift is happening, or if the reasons vary from employee to employee, this could be an indicator that early communication attempts were either ineffective or forgotten.

At this point, benefits advisors and employers should set aside time to recirculate their core messages: why the change is happening, who will benefit from it, when it will happen, what those involved have to do and how they have to do it. It is best to keep these messages short and to the point. Brevity will help ensure they are stored in the memory bank, so when employers ask employees the same questions a few weeks later, the answers should be on point and consistent from one person to the next.

These messages should also be relayed in multiple ways. A face-to-face meeting is a good start, made better when it is followed up with a handout displaying each point and/or an email for individuals to reference later.

Everyone in and connected to the organization – including spouses and other co-beneficiaries – should participate in these discussions and have a clear understanding of the information. Among other things, this will remind employees that this is a group effort, which will only strengthen the alliance for change.

Here is a useful checklist that covers these points:

- Provide a summary of the health plan and vision that is compelling and impossible to misunderstand.
- Include spouses and significant others in communication outreach plans.
- Curate the first patient experience through value-based primary care to bring the communication of the vision to life.
- Create a 12-month editorial calendar of communication that outlines what will be communicated across various channels (email, in-person meetings, posters, etc.).
- Ensure all employee segments, at all levels of the organization, are part of initial and ongoing communications.
- Incorporate feedback loops from employees and spouses as part of the regular cadence of implementation.
- Include primary care partners in member communication.

Step 9: Consolidate Improvements and Build on Gains

Until the new health plan is fully embedded into the organization, the risk of regression remains. Benefits advisors and employers know what kind of barriers to look out for and how to overcome them – especially through communication – but the next step is to really cement progress by consolidating gains and implementing further transformation.

A good indicator that this has happened is when stakeholders, like employees, begin to share the passion. When Jane in IT has a surgery with no copays or deductibles, or when John in Operations can access his care team 24/7, word-of-mouth buzz begins.

Of course, achieving this is easier said than done, and there will inevitably be setbacks along the way. However, there are ways to make sure progress is not undone by complacency.

The first is to always be on the lookout for naysayers. It is quite possible that someone is not thrilled by the health benefits transformation, but – at least for the time being – has decided to go along with it. If their doubts or negative thoughts go on unaddressed, they could quickly fester and spread, waiting to pop up in full vengeance mode when opportunity strikes, as when someone who shares their sentiments finally speaks up.

A small spat of resistance is easier to overcome than an explosion. So, even when things seem to be going well, employers should be watchful. They should never stop asking for feedback, and never stop reiterating important information.

Sometimes individuals will need a little more encouragement. Leaders can offer them just that, through mid-cycle benefits improvement that add even more value to the health plan. Not all of these must be expensive. Here are some examples:

- One employer made free diapers and wipes available for two years for parents choosing the high-value birthing center in their community. Note: The plan was restricted from excluding the price-gouging behemoth health system, so they had to find a creative workaround.
- A professional services firm recognized that the best bill reviewer is the patient and their family. Any plan member who found a billing error the employer would have had to pay received a bonus equal to 20% of the savings. As described earlier, one individual found a $200,000 billing error that the organization was about to pay, and as a result, they received a check for $40,000. After that, no one could ignore how out-of-control many hospital billing practices are.
- A manufacturer added a new Transparent Open Network (TON) benefit and educated employees about how it worked. The contrast shocked them. They saw that most traditional insurers include a PPO discount that does not actually reduce prices, distribute Explanations of Benefits that are incomprehensible, and threaten to send accounts to collections. With the TON, participants started small, using it for just labs and imaging, but eventually saw

that the biggest savings came from surgeries; Before, they would have had a $2,500 out-of-pocket cost, but with the TON, they had zero.

- A large retailer rolled out a cancer-specific concierge service that helped members navigate this difficult treatment and recovery process. With reduced financial and clinical anxiety, these cancer patients had improved health outcomes and significantly lower costs.
- An auto dealer lowered costs and gave employees a month without premiums – an amazing deal that had other auto dealers clamoring for the same success after the story got out.

The lesson: It pays to be proactive and always striving to provide more and better if you want the "new way of doing things" to become the "way we do things around here."

Step 10: Anchor Change into Culture

Cementing change into the culture and preventing the organization from backsliding will require different approaches from one organization to the next, but there are some strategies that consistently work well, including these:

- Discussing the superior results produced by the new benefits approach on a regular basis, clearly explaining the improvement to all stakeholders.
- Incorporating regular updates on health plan progress and setbacks into executive meetings at the highest levels, as well as into leadership and team development meetings.
- Identifying the norms and values that must change to support the new approach.
- Modifying reward programs to align with those new norms and values.
- Counseling, reassigning, or removing employees and managers who are barriers to change and hiring those

whose values and skills match the new norms and values.

- Incorporating education on the new health plan, norms, and values into the onboarding process.
- Supplementing training and development activities to include the skills and competencies required of the new health plan.
- Modifying organizational processes and vendor agreements to align with new norms and values.

These may seem relatively easy to carry out, but they cannot be taken lightly. Culture takes time to develop, and it is only through the consistent execution of these steps that a new culture can take shape and become stronger.

"Time" is a key word here. If employers want to keep newly formed attitudes from fading away, they must accept the fact that they are in this for the long haul. Their actions today, tomorrow, and for the foreseeable future should always be in line with the new company culture, and they should always be working to reinforce it.

Here are a few examples of how employers are doing so:

- One organization publicizes all the money it saves through employee newsletters, posters around the office, monthly savings reports, etc. At the end of the year, it hosts a big party to announce how much the organization saved collectively and highlight how that is going to be reinvested in the business and employees.
- One benefits advisor stresses that all employees have an equity role in the performance of the company, and that every dollar spent on health care is a dollar not spent on their wages or pensions. This approach consistently provides validation and increases employee buy-in.
- Some employers create different contests to hammer home new processes and procedures, bringing some fun into what might otherwise be a boring and tedious information dump.

Key Takeaways and Things to Think About:

- Employers should acknowledge that employees are their most valuable asset and treat them as such. That does not mean tacking on supplemental benefits of low-value, like wellness programs, but designing a health plan that prioritizes value-based primary care.
- Once they understand that, they need to add fuel to the fire by creating a sense of urgency in doing these three things: requesting suspension of disbelief, outlining dysfunction, and making the change effort meaningful by driving home the long-lasting, negative impact of the status quo.
- After the momentum is there, it is essential to have a clear vision on which those undergoing the change can set their sights, based on the organization's own culture/ circumstances. Common vision-setting strategies include the "Nuts and Bolts" Vision, the 11-Star Vision, and the Community-Owned Health Plan Vision.
- Securing grassroots support is the next step. That means starting quietly to build success by having a select few individuals see and experience the new health plan; building from the "bottom" to ensure individuals from each level of the organization are engaged, and educating change agents.
- After the new health plan has been implemented, it is important to sustain change and encourage progress using short-term wins – being on the lookout for and celebrating both the quantitative and qualitative successes the new health plan delivers.
- There will always be pockets of negativity. Here is where leaders should search for signs of structural barriers, psychological barriers, and cultural barriers.
- Leaders must eliminate barriers they identify by talking to both supporters and resisters, thoroughly engaging everyone, implementing change in several stages, and continually communicating change.

- Leaders should always communicate more than they think they need to, checking in on comprehension by asking individuals to explain in their own words what is going on, and revisiting and redistributing the initial messages in various formats – email, posters, in-person meetings, etc.
- In the later stages of the transformation, leaders should still be on the lookout for naysayers, continue to consolidate improvements and build on existing gains, perhaps by making mid-cycle benefits improvements.
- Finally, leaders must make sure they anchor change into organizational culture, or all their efforts will be for naught. That means incorporating health plan values into company values, only hiring and retaining individuals whose skills and attitudes are in line with those new values and making health plan updates/achievements a regular part of the organization's routine.

Additional Background and Resources:

- You Run a Health Care Business Whether You Like It or Not -https://bit.ly/runhcbiz
- 7 Habits of Highly Effective Benefits Professionals -https://bit.ly/benefits7habits

CHAPTER 12

CONCLUSION

After reading this book, I hope you will carry with you these important takeaways:

- We are sinking far too much taxpayer money into health plans and projects that are increasingly and needlessly expensive and fail to produce any added benefit to beneficiaries.
- As a result, other federal, state, and employer initiatives are suffering, negatively impacting education, wages, etc.
- Leaders must adopt an Economic Development 3.0 mindset to turn things around, and benefits advisors and employers must design low-cost, high-quality health plans built on a strong primary care foundation.
- The public, especially millennials, will not settle for anything less. After all, without those two things, we will continue to see spinout public health crises like the opioid crisis.
- A balanced approach must be employed to solve the opioid crisis and the many other issues that stem from our current catastrophic health care system. Doing so requires that we reexamine and readjust how health care is paid for and provided.
- That means looking at and improving the quality of care employees receive with high-cost health plans.

- The best possible health plans keep HEALTH in mind.
- Employers should connect beneficiaries to centers of excellence and not succumb to the wellness program trend.
- Change management is a key part of leading a successful health plan transformation, a process that can be broken down into 10 steps.

Finally, remember this: the key to solving so many Americans' day-to-day frustrations and pain is to slay the health care cost beast. A health care revolution with the intention of doing just that is already underway. In attending this summit and reading this book, you have equipped yourself with the tools you need to join its ranks.

The only question that remains, then, is this: What are you waiting for?

STATUS QUO BENEFITS VS. HEALTH ROSETTA TYPE BENEFITS

Given the massive amount of money spent by employers on health benefits, it's brutal to look at just how bad the status quo is for health benefits. As you review Open Enrollment information, consider that roughly $10,000 is extracted from take-home pay. By comparison, wise employers are spending $5,000-$7,000 per capita with these superior benefits. Reconsider whether you are okay with the status quo. This is even more important, as most employers are going to high-deductible plans and thus what comes out of an employee's paycheck covers less and less. This make health care and health plans one of the few industries where the value proposition gets worse every year. No industry has lower Net Promoter Scores (a measure of customer satisfaction) than Health Plans. Tweaks on the margins won't get the job done.

Status Quo Versus Health Rosetta Comparison

The list of items below gives you a good punch list of what to work on. They are ordered roughly by the level of effort and disruption to the relative payback (i.e., low effort and high ROI bubbles to the top).

Transparent Advisor Relationships

Health Benefits Status Quo	Health Rosetta
"Shops" the insurance every year. Facilitates insurance one year at a time. Believes costs are dependent on the best offer of the carrier. Gives limited data on where your money is going. Provides limited ways to control underlying costs. Doesn't talk about their compensation or worse, is solely paid on commission, meaning more income the broker the more rates go up. Advocates cost-shifting in the form of increased deductibles and copays to lower the employer impact of premium increases Blames costs exclusively on employee behavior and poor health.	· Creates a 3-5-year plan. · Brings transparency to where the money is going. · Talks about their compensation and is willing to tie compensation to performance. · Provides risk management to suit the needs of the business owner(s). · NEVER surprises with a "shock" renewal rate. · Returns control over your costs to you. · Bring the "benefit" of Benefits back to your business. · Makes health benefits a real attraction and retention tool. · Understands *improving* benefits is the only way to lower costs. · Provides detailed data driven analysis and actionable insight.

Active, Independent Plan Management

Health Benefits Status Quo	Health Rosetta
Many ERISA plans have "holes" that expose employers unnecessarily. Pay for high cost ASO networks.	· Fully-compliant ERISA plans that protect companies from abuse. · ERISA fiduciary oversight and review at least as strong as 401k oversight and management. · Use networks focused on high quality providers and geographic coverage.

Transparent Open Networks

Health Benefits Status Quo	Health Rosetta
Wildly variant, opaque pricing for items such as scans, surgeries, and other medical services. If there is any price/quality correlation, it's inversely correlated. Sometimes "transparency" solutions are available giving the best, bad deal while still having co-pays, deductibles, the oxymoronic "Explanation of Benefits," etc. and all the other things that make for a horrible consumer experience.	The good news is there is a solution to the most vexing problem health care has had pricing failure. Fair, fully transparent price to employer/individual at high-quality centers that readily accept quality reporting such as Leapfrog. Providers able to set a price that works for them while avoiding claims/collections hassles and accompanying receivables. No charge for individual going to these providers. No EOBs, bills, etc., just a thank you note.

Value-based Primary Care

Health Benefits Status Quo	Health Rosetta
Flawed reimbursement incentives have turned primary care into "loss leaders" that are like milk in the back of the grocery store (i.e., low margin designed to get people to high-margin items). Short appointments due to not investing properly in primary care. Primary care shortage due to making primary care discipline unappealing. Long wait times to get in can lead to small "fires" blowing up. Medically unnecessary face-to-face appointments clog the waiting room and delay care for people who truly need face-to-face encounters. Record levels of dissatisfaction & burnout amongst PCPs.	· Can fully address over 90% of the issues people enter the health care system for within a primary care setting. · Health coaching addresses lifestyle-driven conditions. · PCP is Sherpa-like resource to help navigate treacherous terrain of complex medical conditions requiring specialty care, procedures, etc. · Same- or next-day appointments for issues not addressed via email/phone. · Extensivist (for the sickest patients) has smaller panel allowing proactive care management & coordination. · Can reduce issues 40-90% and spending 20-50%. · Quadruple Aim leading organizations. · High Net Promoter Scores.

Transparent Pharmacy Benefits

Health Benefits Status Quo	Health Rosetta
Limited or no transparency and control over Pharmacy Benefit Manager (PBM) services. Actual costs often hidden or obfuscated under AWP analysis, rebates, or pseudo-transparency. Including drugs on "preferred" tiers often based on financial, not clinical efficacy, reasons.	· Provide transparency and control over Pharmacy Benefit Manager (PBM) services. · Ensure members have relevant information to make informed choices. · Ensure clinical decisions are based solely on efficacy and ACTUAL cost. · Is a process that works on behalf of the purchaser's best interests.

Benefits Concierge Service

Health Benefits Status Quo	Health Rosetta
Employees left to navigate an extremely siloed and uncoordinated health care system receiving conflicting and often non-evidence-based recommendations.	Having resources to help you navigate the system that can draw on expertise for quality and cost including understanding benefits plans, best provider options, etc.

Major Specialties & Outlier Patients

Health Benefits Status Quo	Health Rosetta
Procedures Quality and prices vary widely. Studies find 40% of transplants are medically unnecessary. High rates of complications at community hospitals who don't do high volumes of complex procedures. **Acute diseases** Little or no evidence-based or patient-specific care or treatment protocols. Highly disjointed care with little communication between providers. No defined approach to match patients to high-quality specialist providers. No access to non-physician resources to facilitate ongoing management or support.	**Procedures** Second opinions at no charge for employee at world-class Centers of Excellence facilities (e.g., Mayo & Cleveland clinics). Unit cost often higher but lower complication rates & avoidance of unnecessary procedures drives strong ROI. Due to the infrequency of these procedures (transplants, neurological procedures, cardiac, spine, and other six-figure or more procedures), this pairs well with Transparent Medical Networks for more common procedures. **Acute diseases** Access to evidence-based and disease-specific care navigation, pathways, and treatment protocols. Highly coordinated care with defined handoffs between care providers. Simple access to high-quality providers with demonstrable strong outcomes. Non-physician care team resources facilitate ongoing management and support.

Appendix

APPENDIX B

A PRACTICAL HANDBOOK FOR SYSTEMS CHANGE

Applied Through Salish|Growth^{src} - A Community Building Company

By Chris Brookfield

"Triggering a widespread economic movement towards decentralization amongst thousands of independent actors."

This handbook describes a process that I have used for 12 years to develop and produce community building companies. In that time, we've recognized a process and shown that it's replicable.

The purpose of this handbook is as an internal resource at Salish | Growth and shared with interested third parties. Salish | Growth focuses on instigating commercial resilience outside of urban cores in the Salish and Columbia Watersheds.

Our work is designed to be entirely open source, and we invite active extension of this work.

Over and over, we have seen that an interdisciplinary approach that joins human focused disciplines with analytical approaches, has triggered large-scale systems change.

Please contact Chris Brookfield (cbookfield@gmail.com) or Arlen Coily (awc468@gmail.com).

O. Introduction to the Nautilus Process

This is a process of system change.

It's nothing new to you.

It has worked for us, over and over.

It can be taught. It can be learned.

Go forward, go backwards, start where you land.

Keep moving.

Systems Change – Establishing Credibility

Unitus Equity Fund - Microcredit for poor communities in India

SKS Microcredit, Bharat (Urban Microcredit)	Microcredit, entrepreneurship, and venture capital led to replication and imitation. Serving millions of families, two of our companies list publicly and one is part of IDFC Bank, a national bank in India.
Ujjivan (Rural Microcredit)	
GVFML (Place Based Microcredit)	

- 10+ million families served
- Over 20,000 jobs created
- Accelerate poor into middle class
- $5+ billion capital crowded in
- 26% Ten Year IRR - cash
- Successful systems change

Elevar - Human centered venture capital develops and funds 20+ human services companies.

Vistaar (Lending to Informal Business)	Twenty human services companies. Grown, replicated, and imitated over and over.
Shubham (Slum Home Improvement)	
Glocal (Rural Acute Health Care)	

- Demonstrates that this process of change can be replicated across diverse services.

North American Grain

Cairnspring Mills (Safe, local, identity preserved flour)	Proof of concept for food system change.

- Demonstrates that this process can be extended to North America.

I. Process

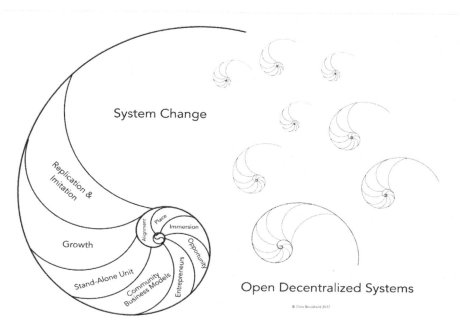

Alignment

Self: Identification of tension between individual/local and legacy/global systems.

Dissonance: Conflict points toward opportunities.

Synthesis: Conflicting values aligned in practice.

Resonance: Community and system values more closely aligned.

Transition: Find a place to practice.

Place

Determine scale: Small enough for local ownership, large enough for economies of scale.

Determine perimeter of focus: Constraints inspire innovative thinking.

Determine identity: Observe social, economic, and geographic organization.

Transition point: Dive into community.

Immersion

Participate: Join community.

Generate empathy: Understand community members.

Build: Personal relationships.

Perceive: Observe, listen, and receive information.

'Map': Social networks.

'Map': Market linkages.

Transition point: Identified essential community needs.

Opportunity

Connect: Needs to resources.

Identify: Barriers and bridges.

Calculate: Potential market size.

Find: Solutions that mimic existing social relationships.

Transition point: *Effervescent community support.*

Entrepreneurs

Rooted: Deeply immersed in community.

Manage: Successful team leader.

Aligned: Active in relevant social movement.

Mindset: Clear vision, open mind.

Transition Point: *Entrepreneur committed to system change for the benefit of their community.*

Community Business Model

Replicate: Models an effective existing relationship in the community.

Iterate: Test and replicate relationship structure.

Gauge: Acceleration of engagement (Suppliers, Clients, Capital) indicates possible model.

Community Support: Facilitates growth and removal of barriers.

Transition: *Defined community business model.*

Stand-Alone Unit

Build: One stand-alone unit

Book: Operational profit

Design: Replicable financial, business, and physical model.

Transition: *Successful imitation & replication.*

Growth

Scale: Grow and add units.

Distribute: Encourage replication & imitation.

Raise capital: Fund expansion, new replication, and new imitation.

Transition: *Business and social movement coalesce and power each other.*

Replication & Imitation

Repeat: Run process again.

Open: Distribute design and process.

Support: Assist in imitation and replication.

Share: Teach and mentor process, encourage imitation.

Transition point: *System changes self-propagate.*

II. Scale

Watersheds

A watershed's boundaries are drawn clearly by mountains, rivers, and floodplains. At this scale, people living in a given watershed share a base of natural resources, culture, and economy. This sharing forms a basis for mutual concern. Watersheds are a natural shape for community formation. Companies may emerge at the watershed scale that reflect the needs of the underlying community. In this way, these companies share local people's pre-existing organization and needs. This partially explains why our companies have historically spent so little on marketing – we do not have to create needs, we do not have to educate consumers about our services, and we do not need to cause community structures to reorient around our distribution.

We have chosen watersheds as our default unit of scale. While we do not know whether a smaller unit, such as a neighborhood, would be better, we do know that just about the entirety of investment management is carried out on much bigger scales. Virtually all money management is national, international, or global in scale. By reducing our scale, we have found solutions and uncovered opportunities that are impossible to see from larger scales.

There appears to be an inherent validity to the watershed scale. Watersheds map very well to the human communities and economies that rest within the physical geography. When we look at these watersheds through history, we find that a great deal of the essential services were defined at this scale. Flour mills were organized by the position of rivers within watersheds. Farmers' fields and agricultural production is organized by watersheds. Towns, cities, and communities are organized by watershed. Much of our work in India was organized into catchments or watersheds.

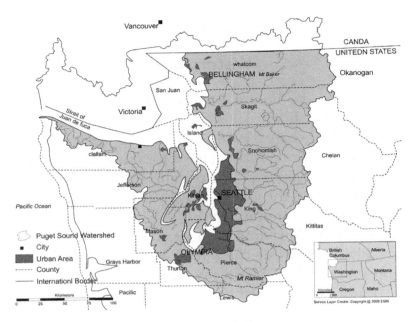

Salish Watershed

One of the insights we discovered at the watershed scale is the remarkable similarity in the network geometry in these watersheds. When the landscape is mapped at this scale, it appears to be a distributed, scale-free network branching out from the river systems. When the community - people and their relationships - are mapped to the watershed, the resultant network is very similar. Both have dense connections in the same areas, around the main stems of rivers. Both are sparse near the steep passes and uplands on the edge of the watersheds. And the amount of market activity mirrors the underlying community and physical geography. In a sense, markets as networks ride atop community and community atop the watershed. Each nested and formed with similar dimensions. Our inquiry into the Skagit River basin, where we found the flour opportunity, reflects this same organization.

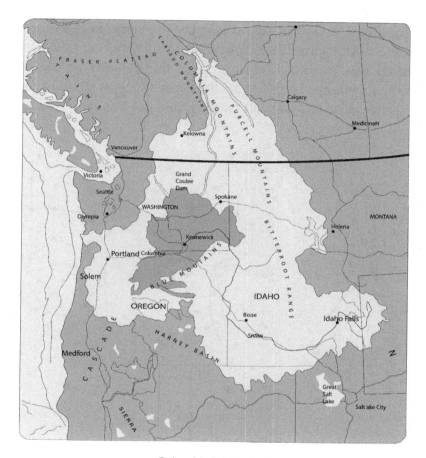

Columbia Watershed

Focus on smaller, more appropriate scales, is one aspect of how we found our flour opportunity and several of our Indian human services opportunities.

Salish | Growth is currently focused on the Salish and Columbia watersheds.

III. Design

We are particularly focused on business models that emphasize *local, open, and independent* attributes. When combined, these attributes create a semi-autonomous distributed network topology.

This topology, or fabric, again reflects the same network geometry as the underlying geography, community and commerce. The design of this business fabric echoes the designs of the nested watershed systems. In this way, the underlying systems – geography, community, and market - strengthen the business model.

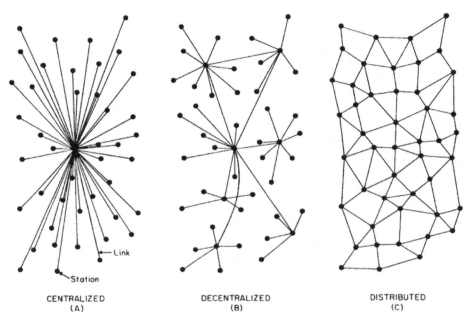

CENTRALIZED
(A)

DECENTRALIZED
(B)

DISTRIBUTED
(C)

Local

By focusing on local, our businesses gain a number of intrinsic advantages that are often overlooked.

First, by decreasing scale, solutions can appear to problems that seem too complicated to solve at global scale. For instance, re-engineering the food system or decreasing poverty really are intractable when viewed at the global scale. Even the basic atoms of these systems, people, are invisible. By dialing into local, new features and relationships emerge. We see that poor people are economically active and can increase productivity with capital access. We see that midscale flour mills can make significant improvements to soil conservation, yields, and overall system resilience, while increasing overall consumer health and satisfaction.

Our local business models are organized in patterns of existing community organization. Our supply chains are short and use existing logistics. Our distribution uses existing networks; we are not attempting to disrupt local relationships. Our services (such as credit, insurance, health care, milling) are considered essential by the community. Because we are offering services that are NOT new, but better mapped to underlying community organization, we need very little money for marketing. We do not need to educate the customer. We do not need to induce changes in community organization. We do not have to pay for engagement. The communities we work in have already done this work for themselves through their social movements.

Open

Our business models are open. This means that we are not even attempting to take proprietary positions or defend our ideas with patents. We share our thinking and discoveries. By being open, each local implementation helps to extend the innovation. Each new watershed can adopt the change through replication and imitation.

Openness is an advantage, largely because information networks have coalesced over the past 15 years and have exponentially increased the flow of information to local communities. There is no way to transmit proprietary ideas at anywhere near the speed and coverage that open sourced ideas move. As information networks have grown, so has the relative advantage in propagating open ideas as compared to contracting proprietary property.

Other than unique names and necessarily personal aspects of our companies, the only aspect of our companies that we protect are the relationships we build. We want to protect and cherish these links to our farmers, bakers, and the community. However, where we have trust and reciprocity, we encourage sharing of relationships, as this speeds replication and imitation.

Independence

Here we mean independence of control, ownership, and production. Since each functional unit is independently owned, there is no central controller. This means that each entrepreneur controls their own brand, production methods, company culture, and resource allocations.

Because our companies are decentralized, they are free to innovate. In flour, we may end up with many variations in how each entrepreneur optimizes their business and serves their customers; choosing their own mill configurations, brands, grain varieties, and growers. By giving up our control as investors, entrepreneurs are put in position to make their own decisions, and the result is a wide diversity of approaches to similar activities. This diversity is at the heart of resilience.

The decentralized business models that are implemented across different watersheds are part of a fabric an interconnected network of autonomous entities. We are not holding proprietary control over the businesses we help start, and we do not intend to be the only ones implementing the nautilus process. We will scale the impact of this company by continuing to replicate the process in new watersheds and new verticals. We will also actively encourage imitation through openness.

As with scale, we are hybridizing our approach to system design to incorporate the best of both local and conglomerated infrastructure. By integrating business models with existing social movements, we achieve network connectivity beyond the local watershed, allowing the sharing of resources, information, and values. By allowing each of these businesses to function autonomously within this fabric and grow to their fullest individual potentials, an individual mill can utilize the control and hierarchical scalability typified by corporation. While at the same time, the fabric, as a whole, achieves quick responses, flexibility, and adaptability – responses which are inhibited by corporate concentration.

THE NATURAL WORLD IS COMPOSED OF DISTRIBUTED ARCHITECTURE

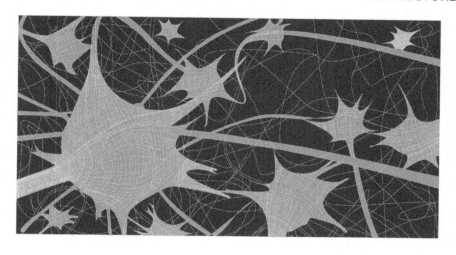

Independent Agents in a Fabric Linked Through Communication

IV. Timing

We have observed that there is a point at which a social movement incorporates the vast majority of people in a community. These movements are very powerful and their power may be expressed through many spheres. Traditionally, social power was viewed as evolving to political power. Through our experience, we have seen that this social power may be directly expressed through market functions.

Our start-ups are fueled less intensely by financial capital and more through the transformation of the underlying social capital. Our companies are built, at their core, to extend, reinforce, and amplify the values represented in the community and the social movement. Our flour mill does well precisely when the values of the local food movement are expressed as consumer behavior. We mirror these values and are supported by them.

Of course, social movements take a long time to gain hold. Finding the right social movement in a specific community with an aligned business model at the right time is the art of this development method and takes patience and experience.

For reference, here are some illustrative timelines for two social movements we have helped develop through community building companies.

Microcredit:

1983 Grameen Bank Founded

2005 UN Year of Microcredit

2006 UEF founded – We initiate investing in microcredit

Mohammad Yunus wins Nobel Prize for microcredit

2014 100 million worldwide borrowers, many public companies

Food System:

1970 First Earth Day

2002 USDA Organic Food Designation Enacted

2010 First Lady Michelle Obama launches healthy food initiative, Let's Move!

2015 Cairnspring Mills established to commercialize healthy, local, and fresh flour

The key here is to acknowledge that movements such as local food and microcredit do not just represent trends. Local food represents the common need for healthy food and unstructured activity, while microcredit represents basic access to capital and human empowerment in poor communities. In these examples, communities have taken into their own hands the instinct and means of change.

One indicator that a movement is ready for development in the commercial sphere is indicated when the movement ceases to be perceived as political within the relevant communities. While movements remain politicized, there is insufficient agreement; when the community itself is split in its support, this method of commercial development is doomed at the outset. On the other hand, it was obvious in the case of both microcredit and local food, that virtually everyone in the local communities agreed with the underlying premise. When the commercial, values-aligned community business models were tested, they were able to attract nearly unanimous support.

Appendix

APPENDIX C

HOW TO PICK A BENEFITS CONSULTANT L

David Contorno

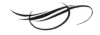

Recently, a Blue Cross health plan offered their brokers a $50,000 reward for switching self-insured clients back to more lucrative, fully-insured plans. In sectors like financial services, that kind of undisclosed conflict could land a person in jail. In health care, however, such clear conflicts of interest are common and considered "business as usual."

For most companies, health care spending is one of the largest expenses on the P&L, often ranking in the top two or three. However, few business leaders give it any more time and attention than they do, say travel or entertainment expenses. Furthermore, some still leave benefits decisions up to the HR department, a seemingly well-intentioned strategy. However, taking an HR-knows-best approach is contrary to the organization's (and often employees') best interests. While HR is critical when it comes to rolling out, administering, and the required employee social counseling of your health plan, financial decisions are best left to officers with an innate ability to negotiate the highly complex.

HR professionals typically fall into one of three categories: coordinator (admin), generalist (social worker), manager (expert). Ruling out the first two as negotiators, expecting your HR manager to deftly navigate a financial win while simultaneously managing recruiting, compliance, compensation, and the entire HRIS system, is akin to finding a unicorn in your driveway tonight. If your broker works closely with HR, and takes your CFO golfing twice a year, he or she is likely paying for the trip with a $50,000 carrier incentive.

Knowing how to select a benefits advisor or consultant* who has the right skill sets and integrity in an industry that is often deliberately opaque can make all the difference in delivering true value to your employees. If you'd like an example of client-first consulting, see the Appendix I "Decoding a fully insured renewal", written by Wes Spencer, an advisor from Michigan.

How We Got Here

Some historical context is important here. In the '70s and '80s, when provider networks were first created, it was generally perceived as a very good thing for the industry and overall health care costs. For the first time, an insurance carrier could negotiate lower, predetermined prices and, in return, drive patients to the providers that agreed to accept these prices.

This allowed carriers to differentiate their networks through the discounts they negotiated with providers, a marketing message that continues to this day. Further, it allowed them to grow market share and, at least in some areas, drive health care financing costs. One thing that didn't change was paying brokers a commission on the premiums of the policies they sell, which dates back to the first life insurance policies sold in the 1800s.

Fast forward to 2010 and the passage of the Affordable Care Act (ACA). One provision, known as the Medical Loss Ratio requirement, was created with good intentions. The premise was that requiring carriers to spend a minimum of 80 to 85 percent of premiums (depending on plan type and employer size) on paying medical claims would prevent them from being overly profitable and would help control costs. It hasn't turned out this way for several reasons. First, after paying medical claims, broker commissions, and normal administrative costs, carriers weren't making an unreasonable profit in the first place. In fact, it is a far smaller percentage of revenue than most businesses would be able to survive on, albeit a small percentage of a VERY large number.

Second, because profit is now tied to a percentage of premium, which is a function of underlying medical costs, the carrier now has an increased financial incentive to ignore rising costs, so long as their costs don't rise any faster than those of their competitors. This certainly existed before 2010, but the ACA turbcharged the dynamic. The common impression that insurance carriers' large networks and client pools give them greater leverage in negotiating prices with providers could not be further from the truth. The more patients a hospital system treats from any particular carrier, the more leverage the hospital system has to increase fees. And employers unwittingly empower the provider's abuse by threatening to leave the carrier if they are unable to come to an agreement to keep that large local health care system in the network, even if it performs poorly.

For many years, all but the very largest employers have been fully invested in this arrangement. Brokers were paid a percentage of premium, employers deferred the entire responsibility for controlling costs to the insurance carrier, individuals consumed whatever care their clinician advised, and everybody was supposedly happy. But as underlying medical costs have gone up, the only winners are the insurance company, care providers (especially hospitals), drug manufacturers, pharmacy benefits managers, and, of course, brokers. [1]

A Broken Process

Here's what typically happens every year for those employers that are fully-insured. We will talk about how this works for self-insured organizations shortly.

Around 60 days prior to the contract renewal date, your broker gets a renewal offer from the current carrier that has VERY little information, explaining the proposed new premiums, which they can now use to shop around the market for a better offer. Note that this market is now tiny. There were 23 national health insurance carriers in 1990; there are now just four.

Let's pause for a moment to consider that the broker often gets no information at all if you have fewer than 100 employees. Even larger employers do not get full transparency, let alone proactive tools to address the underlying medical costs supposedly driving the new, higher rates. If your carrier released more data on your spending, their competitors would be able to "cherry pick" the money-making groups, weeding out the minority that loses them money every year.

Let's assume you are in that minority of money-losing clients. Your carrier has to make you a renewal offer by law. So why wouldn't they just make that offer astronomically high? Because an offer with too large an increase scares off all the other carriers, making it less likely they can get rid of you as a customer, and brings them bad PR to boot.

Playing the Competition

Generally, carriers that want to win your business try to price their offer as high as they can while staying low enough to motivate you to move. That motivation used to be around a 10 percent premium delta, but with costs so high and employers accepting that switching carriers is just part of the game, the delta has shrunk significantly in recent years. Say your initial renewal offer from your current carrier is 18 percent. One of the other carriers believes you'll move for a six percent spread, so they offer a 12 percent increase over your current rates.

If your broker is loyal to your current carrier—and they usually are, because the more clients they have with one car- rier, the bigger their bonus income—he or she will share that 12 percent offer with them. Naturally, that carrier doesn't have to try as hard because they already have your business, so maybe they match the new offer or come in at one percent above or below it.

Some brokers stop right there. They've shown their "value" by reducing the renewal rate by six percent, which can equal hundreds of thousands of dollars in some cases! Plus, you get to keep your current plan and stay with the "preferred" carrier in your state. Oh, and your broker gets a 12 percent pay raise for his efforts—and possibly additional bonus compensation.

Some brokers will send the matching offer back to the other carrier, pitting the two against each other and maybe squeezing out another few points. Either way, your rates are no longer about the cost of your employees' care. They are now about the carriers charging as much as they can while keeping the customers they want. Note that, in the unlikely event your broker was able to save you 20 percent on your premiums, he or she would also take a 20 percent haircut.

The Bottom Line

Once the bottom-line number is reached, if the increase is still more than your budget can handle, the broker will then offer alternative options that inevitably reduce benefits. One impact of reduced benefits has been a dramatic increase in employee out-of-pocket (OOP) costs in recent years, which has made the average worker afraid to even use their plan. Of course, this causes a delay in care until the person is much sicker, creating both a larger claim down the road and additional upward pressure on future rates (not to mention often leaving the employee in a catastrophic financial situation).

One last trick to beware of: Brokers love to wait until the last minute to meet with you to review your upcoming plan renewal. Why? It may be that they are proverbially "fat and happy" and see no need to cater to your needs or perspective. It may be that they have bad news to deliver and prefer to delay tough conversations. Most likely, they feel it will reduce your ability to talk with other brokers and perhaps make a change.

Why do so many brokers support this system? For one thing, it's all they've known. The average age of the typical broker is well into their 50s. For another, as premiums go up, so do their commissions, and carriers offer large bonuses to brokers when they both sell new business and keep the old business where it is. With few exceptions, most states allow for very large "incentive" compensation to brokers. This can mean lavish trips and, more important, as much as a 67 percent increase in pay over the percent paid for the same business to a less loyal broker.

Unless your organization has fewer than 20 people in your health plan, you'd more than likely get great benefits from being self-insured. If your broker/consultant doesn't have that expertise, you are being steered to a plan that benefits the carrier and broker more than you. Many advisors do have that expertise, so be careful about being a guinea pig if the broker has little experience to draw upon.

The No Shop Offer

"David Contorno, because you are such a great partner, we have an amazing offer for our mutual client! If you renew this client without shopping the market, we will come in with an amazingly low renewal AND you will qualify for a $2,500 early renewal bonus! Is this something you would be interested in receiving?"

This is an actual email I, as a benefits consultant, received from a large, well known carrier. It's a tempting offer...I feel like I am in an infomercial of fast talk and supposed deals where all I have to do is act quick and I will get a better deal for me and my client! In my head, I hear the ShamWow guy yelling "If you order in the next 24 hours, we will give you the best deal of your life! But wait, there's more! Act NOW, and we will double your order to include an embedded wellness program, and free telemedicine! But that's not all! We will pay you an additional $2,500! But you must act now!"

Please allow me to translate above... "We at carrier ABC are making so much money on this case, we don't want anyone else possibly exposing that or stealing this nugget of gold from our membership base. Since your expectations of renewals are so low, we don't actually have to price this fairly, all we have to do is come out with a better than expected increase and everyone wins!"

I have to admit, I was seduced by this offer for a long time. I can recall one case, where I was working with my "preferred" carrier at the time, on an existing client. The carrier came to me about 75 days before renewal with a no shop conversation. I asked them where they would be at, absolute bottom line best number, if I agreed to not shop it. They said 5% increase. That seemed extremely reasonable in light of the increases I was getting right around the time when the ACA was being rolled out. When I committed, on my client's behalf (without talking to them) to the offer, I was unaware that the client was already talking to another broker and that broker was out shopping the market. So, I had to backtrack on my "no-shop" promise. The carrier did not like this. The sales manager, to this day, still appears to hold animosity towards me over this case. But here was the outcome...when I was backed into a corner, and had to shop it, the "preferred" carrier of the other broker was coming in exactly in line with the pre-renewal rates. So, I had to push back on the current carrier, completely usurping my promise not to shop it. At the end of the day, we kept the cur- rent carrier and plans, but instead of a 5% increase, we wound up at a 5% decrease... what a great no-shop offer!

Now, if any of you reading this know me, you know this is not a good approach to managing healthcare costs. This is what we as an industry have been doing for decades, and I think the trend speaks for itself. Is a 5% decrease better than a 5% increase? Absolutely.... but when we got this client into a proper self-insured plan about 2 years ago, their costs went down by 41%! And at the same time we reduced out of pocket exposure for most procedures and services to zero for the employee!

The Self-Insured Market

How does this translate to the self-insured market? Most consultants (although not all) who support self-insured plans are far more sophisticated than the brokers profiled earlier. If they're

not, self-insured plans can be a financial disaster of epic propor-
tions. Let's assume this is not the case. A consultant in this space
needs to know (1) how to set up a plan and build it out component by component and (2) how to put protections in place
for your company to ensure your liability is no greater than you
can financially stomach. After all, now you're the insurer and "no
life- time cap" can be a scary proposition. However, a properly
set up self-insured plan actually gives you far more control of
costs than a fully-insured plan. With stop-loss protection, it also
lets you tai- lor your level of comfort with risk.

Here are the main components of high-performing self-insured plans.

- The third-party administrator (TPA) that is responsible for
  paying claims (with your money) according to the speci-
  fica- tions you set up and the supporting plan documents
- The network (usually "rented" from a large carrier) that
  pro- vides "discounts" off billed charges
- Balance billing protection. Employers have a duty under
  ERISA to only pay fair and reasonable charges. After that
  price is determined and paid, some providers will pursue
  an employee to try to get additional payment. A proper
  plan pro- tects employees against this; in extreme cases, it
  can include legal services for the employee.
- A pharmacy manager to handle the pharmacy network
- Pricing contracts
- Stop-loss protection to pay for large claims

So now you are self-insured and are seeing a level of claims
and spending detail you've never seen before. Yet costs are still
going up each year at a similar rate, or maybe you saved some
money the first couple of years. But now what? This is where the
rubber meets the road for the more advanced consultant.

A common first misstep to lower costs is workplace wellness programs. As we saw in *Are Workplace Wellness Programs
Hazardous to Your Health?* at best, only a tiny percentage of such

programs have a real ROI. At worst, they can cost a bunch more money while irritating and potentially actually harming your employees. At least, in the self-insured environment, you have access to data that can point you toward risk factors to focus on (or scuttle the entire program). But the initial excitement and enthu- siasm over data access and your fancy new workplace wellness program quickly dies. Seventy-two percent of companies have these programs and, I assure you, Seventy-two percent of companies are not happy with their health care spending trends.

Instead, a progressive consultant brings you a multiyear health care plan designed to lower the price and use of overtreatment, which harms employees financially and potentially medically. The plan is built on a proven approach to lowering the actual cost of care for ALL employees, whether they are healthy or not, and will generally reflect the following:

- Serious thought for ERISA fiduciary responsibility
- An emphasis on value-based primary care
- An emphasis on the highest-cost outlier patients
- Transparent open networks/reference-based pricing (i.e., ways to know the actual prices you'll pay for services)
- Transparent pharmacy benefits
- Data proficiency

The plan will also include payment arrangements with providers and, importantly, complete disclosure of the consultant's sources of compensation.

Value Counts More Than Fees

However, none of this can take place if your company makes one very common mistake: selecting a consultant at the same time you select your plans and other benefits for the upcoming year. A forward-looking consultant will help you see these as two distinct decisions that should be made at separate times.

As you can see, the actual "insurance" is a smaller and smaller piece of what the nontraditional benefits consultant brings to the table. In the self-insured model, stop-loss is the only insurance policy purchased, generally accounting for less than 20 percent of overall costs. Your consultant should be able to provide you with all the information you need to identify the best renewal options for noninsurance administrative functions and, critically, the right strategies to positively impact both the cost and quality of your employees' care over the long term.

You don't necessarily want to pick your consultant based on how low their fee is. (Fees are usually a small percentage, in the low single digits, of your total health care spend, which doesn't speak to their true value.) This is how most businesses make that decision, and we all know how well that's been working. A truly innovative consultant will be willing to put some of their compensation at risk, based on performance, and turn the commission conundrum described earlier on its head. Imagine paying your consultant more based on money actually saved! Now that's aligning incentives.

While no one expects an organization leader to be an expert in all these areas, you should be generally aware enough to ensure that the people trusted with handling one of your largest expenses are. Pick your benefits advisor with greater care than you would pick a 401-k advisor. After all, not only is there the same ERISA fiduciary liability as 401-k plans, a status quo plan can subject your employees to unnecessary medical harm. One way you can judge a consultant's skill, integrity, and expertise is whether they're certified by the Health Rosetta. Certification requires transparency, expertise in key areas and strategies, and adherence to valid cost and outcome measure- ment models. Many seasoned, high integrity professionals have already received this qualification. Learn more at healthrosetta.org/employers.

David Contorno is a nationally recognized speaker, author and founder of E Powered Benefits which helps employers and brokers to lower costs and improve outcomes.

Key Takeaways

- If your health care costs have increased over the course of the last 5 years, there is a good chance you need a new advisor.
- Separate the annual benefits process from the benefits advisor decision by as much time as possible.
- Beware of brokers unwilling to align your financial interests with theirs. At the same time, value counts more than fees, so avoid being penny wise and pound foolish.

Appendix

APPENDIX D

CLIENT NOTICE, PLAN SPONSOR BILL OF RIGHTS, AND CODE OF CONDUCT

Sample Health Rosetta Client Notice

Congratulations! We're excited you've decided to work with a Health Rosetta Certified Benefits Professional. The Health Rosetta ecosystem's mission is to help group benefits purchasers sustainably reduce health benefits costs and provide better care for their employees. We maintain the Health Rosetta, an expert sourced blueprint for wisely purchasing benefits sourced from the highest-performing benefits purchasers and experts everywhere.

A primary goal of Health Rosetta certification programs is to help benefits purchasers reduce your spending while improving the quality of care your plan members receive. This notice is to help you understand what to expect working with a Health Rosetta Certified Benefits Professional.

What to Expect?

One of our core principles is that higher transparency, trust, and integrity in the purchasing process improves the quality of benefits-purchasing decisions. To facilitate this, HRI certified professionals commit in our agreement with them to adhere to certain specific practices.

- Only make changes that have been shown to improve care while improving your costs AND your employees' costs. No more choosing between hurting you or hurting your employees.
- Review this notice with you to set expectations.
- Fully and meaningfully disclose their compensation in writing.
- Think, plan, and act in your long-term interests, including completing 3-5-year strategic plans.
- Adhere to the HRI Code of Conduct you should have received with this notice
- Adhere to the HRI Plan Sponsor Bill of Rights you should have receive with this notice.

These practices significantly differentiate both certified professionals and their design, purchasing, and management process from the highly-conflicted, opaque status quo process. To maintain the quality of HRI certification programs, they'll ask you to sign this notice and a couple other documents throughout the purchasing process.

How the Health Rosetta Ecosystem and Certification Benefit You

You'll likely benefit both directly and indirectly as a result of working with a HRI-certified benefits professional. Here are a couple of the main ways.

- Higher-value benefits – You should start seeing returns in the form of sustainably lower costs and higher quality care within the next 12 months. While we can't promise specifics, as this varies on many factors, Health Rosetta components implemented by other employers have sustainably reduced their spending by 10-40% per year.

- Access to a deep ecosystem of solutions and best practices – Our health care system is in the early days of a dramatic transformation, with many new innovative approaches. This makes it difficult for you and most advisors to see through the noise. Certified professionals have access to other certified people, industry leading experts, the Health Rosetta blueprint, and other community resources to sift through this, improving the likelihood that design changes, programs, technologies, and services you implement are appropriate and likely to work.

- Learning from others – The education and other resources we make available for certified professionals are based on the real-life experience of other purchasers, not theory. We actively cultivate shared learning to keep us abreast. We maintain a network of more than 3,500 experts and high national visibility to create a hivemind for identifying the best approaches. See just a few of our collaborators at healthrosetta.org/whowe-are/.

We have high expectations for certified professionals and work to attract those seeking to go above and beyond them. However, if you feel your certified professional is not meeting your needs, discuss with them or contact us directly at employers@healthrosetta.org. We're happy to help. You can find more resources, our book, *The CEO's Guide to Restoring the American Dream*, and subscribe to updates and education at healthrosetta.org.

From Dave, Sean, and the entire Health Rosetta team, we'd like to thank you for choosing to work with a HRI-Certified Professional.

Health Rosetta Plan Sponsor Bill of Rights

1. Service Agreement Fiduciary Duty Protection

You have the right to ensure that your obligations as your plan's sponsor, administrator, and fiduciary are protected and enhanced in your service agreement.

2. Transparent Relationships & Conflict Disclosure

You have the right to expect transparency, including disclosure of conflicts, in financial dealings between you and your broker, advisor, or consultant, carriers, and vendors.

3. Independence

You have the right to ensure those financial dealings do not compromise your fiduciary responsibility and the independence of the advice you receive.

4. Access to all options

You have the right to receive information about the full range of options available to you, not just those that preserve or optimize your representative's income or plan administrator's revenue.

5. Independent Review

You have the right to an unbiased, independent review of all pertinent market options in an impartial manner, not just those that preserve or optimize your representative's income or plan administrator's revenue.

6. Comprehensive Reporting

You have the right to receive comprehensive reporting of your costs, and the potential drivers of those costs.

7. Answers to Questions

You have the right to receive answers to your questions, with no cloaking of responses with HIPAA Privacy and other "confidentiality" curtains.

8. Effective Adjudication

You have the right to expect those you hire to adjudicate benefits to give their best effort to identifying inappropriate and grossly inflated charges before they issue payment.

9. Access to data

You have the right to your data and should agree upon this requirement prior to execution of any vendor agreement.

10. Complete reporting

You have the right to receive complete service and outcome reporting from each of your vendors, including all fees associated with services rendered.

Health Rosetta Benefits Advisor Code of Conduct

Good for employees and employers

We resolve to only implement programs and solutions that seek to improve the plan sponsor's bottom line, the plan member's bottom line, and, most importantly, the plan member's health.

Programs should do no harm

We resolve that brokers, consultants, and advisors should do no harm to employee health, corporate integrity, or employee/employer finances. Instead, we will endeavor to support employee well-being for our customers, their employees, and all program constituents.

Employee Benefits and Harm Avoidance

We will only recommend implementing programs with/ for employees rather than to them, and will focus on promoting responsible practices for the health plans we serve.

Our choices of programs and strategies shall always prioritize best outcomes at the lowest cost, in that order, with a strong focus on the responsibility that an employer should provide affordable coverage for their employees while respecting the financial integrity of the business.

Respect for Corporate Integrity and Employee Privacy

We will not share employee-identifiable data with employers and will ensure that all protected health information (PHI) adheres to HIPAA regulations and any other applicable laws.

Commitment to Transparency

Our focus shall be to bring transparency to all levels of health care financing. From how we get paid to how insurance companies and PBMs get paid to how providers get paid.

Commitment to Valid Outcomes

Measurement of contractual language and outcomes reporting will be transparent and plausible. The end goal is to improve outcomes and quality of care while lowering costs, and the ability to do this shall be measured and reported on in a valid, consistent, and accountable format.

APPENDIX E

SAMPLE COMPENSATION DISCLOSURE FORM

The following is a sample broker compensation disclosure form to help you improve your benefits purchasing process. The status quo is rife with conflicts of interest stemming from undisclosed compensation arrangements. This prevents benefits purchasers from making the most informed and intelligent purchasing decisions. We've found that the first step toward high-performance benefits is disclosure of incentives to minimize conflicts, create transparency, and increase trust in your advisors and process.

Calculation of Fees

In general, each fee should be calculated in one of five ways.

1. **Premium based.** Fees are based on the amount of premium for each line of coverage. This is normally expressed as a predetermined percentage.
2. **Claims-based.** Fees are based on the $ amount or number of claims in the plan and generally are expressed as percentages or aggregate per-claim fees for the period.
3. **Per member or eligible employee (e.g., PMPM/PEPM).** Fees are based on the number of eligible employees or actual members in the plan.

4. **Transaction-based**. Fees are based on the execution of a particular plan service or transaction.
5. **Flat rate**. Fees are a fixed charge that does not vary, regardless of plan size

You can also access a regularly updated digital version of this firm on the Health Rosetta Institute's website (healthrosetta.org).

HEALTH ROSETTA INSTITUTE BENEFITS
REPRESENTATIVE COMPENSATION DISCLOSURE
FORM

Advisor: _____   Client: _____   Period: _____

Background

A key element of the Health Rosetta Institute's mission is to help benefits purchasers build transparent, trusted relationships with benefits advisors. These relationships are critical to an effective benefits-purchasing process, particularly in today's world of skyrocketing health care costs and limited ability to push those costs on employees. This form is one resource to help you.

Advisor compensation is a small portion of total spend, but the right one can guide the way to dramatic improvements in your plan costs and quality. The total amount shouldn't be the primary focus. Instead, it should help build trust and identify potential conflicts.

High-value, forward-leaning advisors are worth their weight in gold. Plus, the strategies they use typically improve your bottom line, reduce your employees' out-of-pocket spending, and improve the quality of care they receive. Think of it this way:

Would you rather pay four percent to an advisor who reduces total spending by 15 percent or two percent to one who "negotiates" a 15 percent increase down to a seven percent increase? For every 100 employ-

ees on an average plan, you'd save $247,220 in year 1 and $1.2 million in 5 years (net of the higher compensation).

Unwillingness to disclose compensation is typically a red flag that recommendations may not align with your interests. The benefits world often has undisclosed conflicts and incentives that make intelligent purchasing decisions difficult. To help you get around this, we've created a free guide for selecting high-value advisors.

Contact us at healthrosetta.org to learn more about improving the cost and quality of your health plan, about Certified Professionals, and about how we help benefits purchasers. A special thanks to Eric Krieg at Risk International Benefits Advisory, David Contorno at Lake Norman Benefits, Josh Jeffries at Arkin Youngentob Associates, and Tom Emerick at Edison Health for helping create this form. Each is a worth-their-weight-in-gold type.

Overview of Services Provided

Some fees may be estimates and will vary throughout the course of the year. However, the variance shouldn't be significantly, unless something significant and unplanned happens.

Service Provided	External Vendor	Cost/ Fee for Service	Compensation Type	Total Compensation
Core Consulting Services				
Pharmacy Consulting Services				
Actuarial Services				
Compliance Services				
Wellness Consulting				
Claims Audit				
Data Analytics and Clinical Services				

Communications				
Decision Support Services and Transparency Resources				
Benefits Administration				
Total Projected Annual Costs				

Expected Financial Compensation from External Vendors

Category	Vendor	Effective Date	Compensation Type	Total Compensation
Medical				
Rx				
Dental				
Vision				
Stop loss				
EAP				
FSA				
Group Life				
AD&D				
LT Disability				
ST Disability				
Cancer				
Critical Illness				
Wellness				
Disease Mgmt.				
Broker Fee				
Other				
Total				

Are any compensation multipliers or other bonuses applicable to the above categories of compensation?
☐ Yes (please describe below)   ☐ No

If yes, are they included in the above dollar amounts?
☐ Yes   ☐ No

Do you or your firm accept any non-account specific financial compensation from any products, services, or vendors you're recommending, including, but not limited to, contingent or bonus commissions, override or retention bonuses, and backend commissions?
☐ Yes (please describe below)   ☐ No

Do you or your firm have any other financial or non-financial compensation, potential conflicts of interest, or incentives related to products, services, or vendors you're recommending, including, but not limited to, ownership, equity stakes, revenue/profit sharing, GPO/coalition participation, preferred vendor panels, conferences or trips, or personal relationships?
☐ Yes (please describe below)   ☐ No

Are there any potential reasons that could cause costs of services or compensation to vary more than 10 percent from the above projections?
☐ Yes (please describe below)   ☐ No

Please describe details related to any questions to which you answered yes above, including the specific, expected, or estimated dollar value. Attach additional pages if necessary.

Total Expected Compensation

Consulting Services	
Compensation from External Vendors	
Cost of Services from External Vendors	

Advisor

I certify that to the best of my knowledge the above is a complete and meaningful disclosure of my firm's entire compensation.

Client

I acknowledge that the signed Certified Advisor has presented and adequately reviewed the above disclosures.

Name: _____

Entity: _____

Title: _____

Signed: _____

Date _____

Name: _____

Entity: _____

Title: _____

Signed: _____

Date _____

APPENDIX F

HEALTH ROSETTA PRINCIPLES

The Health Rosetta Principles were created and curated with Leonard Kish. We drew these insights from dozens of the most forward-looking individuals in the health care industry. The Health Rosetta components in part IV of the book speak to how health care purchasers can be wise about their health care purchasing. The principles below speak to how the health care industry should respond to changing purchasing and patient behavior to navigate uncharted terrain. They are the guide for how the industry can succeed in the future health ecosystem.

Leading thinkers ranging from Bill Gates to Esther Dyson have written essays on specific principles that we invite you to read at healthrosetta.org/health-rosetta-principles. The essays expand on each principle to make them more actionable. In the open-source spirit of the Health Rosetta, we invite others to contribute their essays to advance the cause.

A New Medical Science

1. *A New Paradigm* – A new social, psychological, biological, and information-driven medical science is emerging that will better understand a person's environmental context and its relationship with disease. It's precision medicine but more, using sensors and networks to better predict and prevent as well as treat

the root causes of disease. No vision of the future of medicine can be complete or even competent if it doesn't recognize these new sources of information and the power of patient engagement.

2. *Open source and open knowledge* – Open source, open APIs, open data, and open knowledge (such as wikis) will become central to defining a common architecture to support this new science. These are modern versions of peer review.

3. *Nonclinical determinants of outcomes* – To improve care and reduce costs with this new science, we must focus on what drives 80 percent of outcomes, the nonclinical factors, which include social, economic, and psychological determinants of health.

4. *Cross-disciplinary collaboration* – Cross-disciplinary collaboration and sharing of research data will be a requirement to accelerate new discoveries.

5. *Evidence-based understanding of what works* – This new science will arrive at an evidence-based understanding of what works through a great wealth of shared longitudinal health data captured through mobile devices, sensors, and health records. It must be mindful of the concept of transforming data to actionable information, knowledge, and wisdom.

6. *Understanding the personome* – The new medical science will focus on understanding the personome. "The influence of the unique circumstances of the person—the personome—is just as powerful as the impact of that individual's genome, proteome, pharmacogenome, metabolome, and epigenome."

Openness Drives Effective Action

7. *Individual choice* – Individuals have the right to make choices and control their health destiny with the best information available.

8. *Open access to information* – Open access to information will enable individuals to make the best decisions and become well-informed individuals, particularly when curated and contextualized by clinicians.

9. *Openness and privacy are not in conflict* – Openness and privacy are not in conflict with the right kinds of identity, consent, and data-control mechanisms in place.

10. *A required culture change* – This openness will come with a required culture change. We must release information in order to ensure high-quality information and code. In software, Linus' Law states, "Given enough eyeballs, all bugs are shallow." Keeping information sealed until it is perfect will mean we miss opportunities to improve the data and fix the system.

Economics and Transparency

11. *Information asymmetries* – Information asymmetries lead to inefficient systems and suboptimal outcomes. Access to life-saving, taxpayer-supported research must be open.

12. *Social determinants of health* – Health and wealth are tightly linked. Eventually, poor financial health will negatively impact overall health.

13. *Cost as comorbidity* – The cost of care can be a comorbidity. By ignoring costs in clinical decisions, conditions can worsen as financial stress may drive individuals to choose not to follow a plan of care because it is too expensive.

14. *Individual's right to know the cost of care* – Individuals have the right to know how much care will cost before receiving care, whether that cost is out-of-pocket or covered. When there is unpredictable complexity (not caused by medical error, which shouldn't be charged for at all), individuals should be informed of the most likely ranges.

15. *Personal responsibility* – Individuals have personal responsibility to manage their lives along with their care.

Relationships and Peer-to-Peer Networks Will Become Central

16. *Communication as medical instrument* – The most important

"medical instrument" is communication. Communications drive actions, build relationships, and create trust.

17. *Data liquidity for improving health* – Exchange of personal health data will become enabled via decentralized Peer-to-Peer (P2P) networks and "HIEs of 1." These P2P exchanges will improve health literacy, healthy action, and a functioning health economy.

18. *P2P networked conversations* – P2P networked conversations will empower new ways of better organizing health, allowing individuals to "organize without organizations" (h/t Clay Shirky) for better care.

19. *Individuals and health research* – Verifiable but deidentified, opt-in health data will become part of a unified view for research and risk assessment. Individuals will have the choice to contribute.

New Intelligence

20. *Cognification* – To "Cognify" (h/t Kevin Kelly) is to instill intelligence into something. Medical knowledge will increasingly be "cognified" into the IoT as much of the world around us is made "smart" and data-aware. This is good and will free people to care for themselves where and when they choose.

21. *Feedback* – All feedback has utility. Whether the news is good or bad, opinions that become known are a source for improvement and competitiveness.

Community-driven Health

22. *Stewarding social and economic factors* – True health system leadership comes from not just being stewards of hospitals and clinics but stewarding social and economic factors and the physical environment of a community, which account for half of outcomes.

23. *Partnering for community health* – Assessing community health

needs and adopting strategies to address those needs will provide hospitals with a valuable opportunity for community partnerships to identify strategies for improving health, quality of life, and the community's vitality.

24. *Building health literacy and community* – Health care organizations that aggressively promote health literacy will build community capacity in addressing health issues. This may mean enabling and curating others in the community to reach everyone.

25. *Health and financial literacy* – Start by teaching medicine and psychological self-awareness and resilience to kids. Health education should include the "medicine" we consume every day (i.e., food). Insurance/benefits literacy should be included in schools' financial literacy courses.

26. *School lunches* – School lunches are an access point of great power: they reinforce or remove the unhealthy products we consume.

27. *"Let food be thy medicine"* – Hippocrates said, "Let food be thy medicine and medicine be thy food." Individuals are "poisoning" themselves with the food they eat, largely without knowing it.

28. *"Walking is man's best medicine."* – Hippocrates also said, "Walking is man's best medicine." Communities and workplaces that make it easy to walk and be active can gain an advantage over the status quo.

29. *Health care waste: A bandit stealing from our future* –Health care is breaking U.S. schools. Money once directed to education is getting gobbled up by health care's hyperinflation, exacerbating the problem that kids don't learn enough about health, nutrition, finance, or any of the things that lead to healthy, long lives.

New Choices for Individuals and Care Teams

30. *Health isn't limited to the clinic* – Health is not the limited time individuals spend in clinics. What happens in the other 99+ percent of their life has the greater impact on an individual's overall well-being.

31. *Better choices through motivation* – We will learn how to rapidly enable better choices through motivation, tools, and access to better choices and lifestyles. Each individual will respond differently, requiring a whole new level of personalization.

32. *Understanding motivations and habit change* – People are complicated with both innate drives and ingrained habits that work against long-term health. The psychology of understanding these motivations and habits is critical to success in achieving better health.

33. *Wisdom of the individual* – People will make incredibly smart decisions when they understand the true risks and choices.

34. *Mental health* – Mental health is an equal component of a person's overall health. Mental health directly impacts our physical health and our ability to recover from disease or medical interventions. Therefore, mental health needs to be deliberately and systematically integrated into the general health care system.

35. *Nutritional and environmental causes of disease* – Open information and research are needed to understand the nutritional and environmental causes of disease.

36. *Unhealthy food* – Foods that are devoid of nutrition are the tobacco of this generation.

37. *Optimizing health* – We have defined sick care very well: what happens when things go wrong and how to correct them. We have very little understanding of how to keep things going right, how to get people back on track when they go off the rails, or how to continually optimize health. Innovations in research are changing this; new entrants will figure out how to enable it.

38. *Preventing the need for care* – Systems will be designed so indi-

viduals can stay healthy, take as few drugs and have as few procedures as possible, and avoid the system as much as possible by engaging in self-care.

39. *Embracing the "flat world" of care* – The emergence of a flat world opens new avenues to innovation around what has worked in other cultures. We have the opportunity to learn to be open to ways of health care that originate outside our borders, particularly those that are more appropriate to the underserved.

Individuals and Engagement

40. *Inclusivity with individuals and caregivers* – Individuals and their everyday caregivers are the greatest untapped sources of information, knowledge, and motivation. Empowering them to work together will optimize care.

41. *Experience had a "Triple Aim" too* – The effectiveness of engagement is tightly aligned with how convenient it is; how easily it integrates with where we live, work, and play; and how culturally relevant and cost-effective it is.

42. *Leveling the playing field* – Engagement and empowerment are different. Individuals are often most engaged, but least empowered. Putting individuals and clinicians on the same level will improve care.

43. *"Patient engagement" is backwards* – "Patient engagement" is valuable but backwards. Individuals need the health system to be engaged with them and regularly, not just during visits.

44. *"Individual-centered" engagement* – An engaged individual is very different from "patient engagement" (h/t Gilles Frydman). One is individual-centered, one is health system-centered. Achieving full health is the goal, not engaging with the health system.

45. *Engagement for avoiding the health system* – An individual can be engaged with their own health without entering the health system at all (h/t Hugo Campos), and this is a good thing.

New Economics

46. *Choose wisely* – Oftentimes, less is more.
47. *Prevention* – Oftentimes, early is better than late.
48. *Overtreatment* – Overtreatment is one of health care's greatest challenges. In many cases, no treatment is much better than treatment.
49. *Sustainability* – A system that profits more from people with "problems" than those without and has a default set at "treat more" is destined to collapse due to its inherent unsustainability.
50. *Evidence-based care delivery* – Driven by individual's access to information and, informed by statistics, treatment will become better aligned with science.
51. *Empowering a patient to make rational economic choices* – Individuals enter the health care system to get measurements; to be diagnosed; and to seek answers and, when appropriate, treatment. Individuals who can will increasingly seek alternatives outside of expensive, inconvenient care centers. This will drive positive overall change in the health system.

New Education

52. *Scaling medical education for the future* – Medical education will be made continuous, engaging, and scalable in the age of increasing clinical demands and limited work hours.
53. *New approaches to learning* – Medical educators will make thoughtful use of technology and learning design. Those who excel will learn how MOOCs, community engagement, social media, simulation, and virtual reality can enhance medical education.
54. *Harnessing the data deluge* – The flood of new medical information is impossible for any one person to stay on top of. Physicians and other care providers will be enabled by better systems for filtering what's valuable for an individual's care.

55. *Rapid evolution* – Effective medical education must and will evolve rapidly to focus on care delivery and the use of digital tools in care delivery.
56. *Physician as community manager* – Medical education will recognize that, because only 10–20 percent of health outcomes are driven by clinical care, physicians must also be stewards of community transformation, entering into multidisciplinary alliances.

New Data Ownership Rights

57. *Individual Rights* – An individual's access to and management of data about him/herself is a fundamental human and property right. Why is it easier to have your medical data hacked than for you to get access to it? (h/t Eric Topol)
58. *Monopolies* – Monopolies on medical knowledge and information are unethical.
59. *Single Patient Record* – Now that all information can be connected all the time, there should be only one record of health data that comes from an individual, controlled by the individual. Problems with HIPAA and "information blocking" are symptoms of a broken, pre-Internet, paper-driven era.
60. *Property Rights in a Distributed System* – Platforms will be developed to enable transactions around health data property that are decentralized, yet able to focus on the individual in an instant. Be prepared.
61. *Patients' Right to Data About Them* – Individuals have a right to any data that comes from measuring an internal state of their body, including from medical devices.
62. *Immediacy of Access to Health Data* –People have literally died, waiting for their lab data. Lab and other data should be made accessible to the individuals as soon as it is available.
63. *Data Doesn't Cause Medical Harm* – Medical regulations exist to protect individuals from medical harm. Data, ideas, and information in the hands of individuals cause no medical harm.

64. *Safe Access to Data Without a Doctor's Permission* – Individuals should have access to metrics and analysis about their own body without a doctor's permission as long as that access poses no significant medical risk.

65. *Right to Privacy* – Individuals have a right to health data privacy and only they or their legal agent can give permission for sharing their data.

66. *Health Information Anti-Discrimination* – Health data collected about an individual cannot be used to determine a person's access to capital (via credit ratings), employment, education, housing, or health care services. This will be legislated and ensured by new technologies.

New Roles and Relationships for Providers

67. *Misaligned Incentives* – Misaligned reimbursement schemes have impaired providers from doing the primary job of healing and have often robbed them of their humanity. Paying for value will help them reverse course.

68. *Enlightened Providers Partner with Patients* – The enlightened clinicians who embrace these guiding principles will gain a powerful competitive advantage by partnering with patients who have taken responsibility for their own care.

69. *Maintain Trust in Health Professionals* – Nurses, doctors, and pharmacists are among the most trusted professionals; they need to respect this trust and continue to earn it by influencing patients only for the patients' good.

70. *Whole-Person View of Health* – World class care teams require a holistic view of a person's complete health, which includes their mental health as well as their physical health.

71. *Embracing the Science of Behavior Change* – Relationships fuel behavior change (both positive and negative); motivation, triggers, and ease of action are keys to enabling that change.

72. *The Importance of Relationships* – Aim to motivate, teach, consult, and enable. Clinicians cannot expect participation in a care plan (i.e., "adherence") without mutual understanding. Recognize

that when an individual is not incapacitated, they are in control of whether they fill prescriptions, follow a care plan, etc.

73. *Health Care Extends Beyond the Walls of the Clinic* – The best care is and will be collaborative beyond the walls of any one institution. Just as "the smartest people work for someone else," the smartest providers practice outside of one clinic or hospital. The smartest provider may, in fact, be a collective, or the crowd. New ways to open communications will drive better care.

74. *Flipping the Clinic* – Many times, the best place for interaction between the clinician and an individual isn't at the clinic. We can flip the clinic. Much of what has been done at a clinic visit can be done more effectively in the comfort of an individual's home via email and other digital tools or in social settings such as churches or community organizations.

75. *Embracing Data to Deliver Better Care* – The most relevant providers will be conversant with data analytics and tools. They will be experts in care delivery, not just diagnostics and traditional medical science.

A New Competition in Life Science & MedTech

76. *Embracing the New Science* – Tomorrow's leaders will redesign research and development to capitalize on new science dynamics and mobile technologies.

77. *Embracing New Partnerships* – New and nonobvious partnerships will need to be forged to ensure leadership in the future. Alliances with health tech and consumer health Internet companies will be as important as alliances with academic medical centers have been in the past.

78. *Broadening the Value of Post Research Relationships* – Posttrial relationships with individuals will allow cocreation and insights not possible before. That is a largely untapped opportunity. ResearchKit is just the beginning.

79. *Openness to Engagement* – The individual's relationship to a device or therapeutic may be as profound as their relationship to their doctor, or more so. Be available and open to such engagement to make improvements.

New Health Plans, New Health Benefits

80. *Fee for Service Is Dying* –Transition now in every way you can.
81. *The Dirty Secret of Health Plans* – The dirty secret of health plans is that higher care costs have, counterintuitively, led to greater profits for the plans. This is changing. Winning health plans will capitalize on the opportunity to fundamentally rethink plan design to be optimized for the fee-for-value era.
82. *Catalyzing Patient Engagement* – Catalyzing patient engagement will lead to better care and a more competitive offering.
83. *The Next Dirty Secret* – The next dirty secret of health plans is that they are money managers. The longer they hold onto money, the more they make.
84. *Investing in Members' Financial Security* – Rather than reflexively denying claims and building up a mountain of ill will, insurance companies should invest resources in protecting their member's financial security.
85. *The "Negaclaim"* – Customers will, in effect, "self-deny" their own claims. A new metric for success is the "Negaclaim"—an unnecessary claim avoided. This isn't about denying care. Just as energy consumers aren't interested in kilowatt hours, individuals aren't interested in health claims—they want health restored and diseases prevented.
86. *True Informed Consent* – When individuals are fully educated on the trade-offs associated with interventions, they generally choose the less invasive approach.
87. *"Essential Access," the Corollary to "Essential Benefits"*—The ACA defined "essential benefits" but there will be a corollary about rights to "essential access" as part of coverage. Any modern health plan offering will include virtual visits, transparent price info, updated provider directory, same-day

e-mail response, next-day test results, etc.—all eminently doable with today's modern technology.

88. *Rethinking Benefits Design and Procurement* – As CFOs & CEOs are failing in their fiduciary responsibility by being overly passive in how they procure health benefits, the second or third biggest expense after payroll. A rethought health care purchasing plan drives direct financial returns, but, most importantly, enables your valued employees to do what they desire—realize their full potential. Elements are defined at healthrosetta.org.

89. *Aligning Laboratory Testing and Genomics* – Genomics and proteomics information and testing will be key components of personalized medications, tailored to provide the best dose/ response relationship in each patient. Because of their importance, these tests and genomic information must be covered by health plans and insurance.

New Health System

90. *Transitioning Care Beyond the Walls of the Clinic* – Hospitals have provided amazing service for the last 100 years, but location is becoming less important for health care. Care can happen almost anywhere at lower cost. What conditions hospitals treat, and how hospitals serve their communities will dramatically change over the coming decades.

91. *Reimagining Technology in the Fee-for-Value Era* – Health systems' technology procurement process must be up to the task. Systems grown and optimized for the waning fee-for-service era often have the polar opposite design to what will optimize the fee-for-value era. Virtually every new health care delivery organization that is outperforming on Triple Aim objectives has deployed new technology reimagined.

92. *Focusing on Communication over Billing* – Outside of health care, millions of organizations have reformulated how they interact with their ultimate customers with better communications tools. Next generation health care leaders understand that tools will focus on communication over billing.

93. *Borrowing a Page from the Newspaper Industry* –Newspaper executives dismissed an array of new asymmetric competitors including eBay, Craigslist, Monster.com, Cars.com, Facebook, Groupon, ESPN, CBS Marketwatch and more who stole advertising, media consumption, or both. Health system executives are doing the same thing today, and the issue is the same: how valuable content will be delivered in the future. The content is different, but the issue of distribution is the same.

94. *The "Forgotten" Fourth Aim* – Winning health care delivery organizations recognize that the Quadruple Aim will deliver sustainable success. The "forgotten aim" is a better experience for the health professional, which leads to a better experience and better outcomes for patients. Layering more bureaucracy on top of an already overburdened clinical team ignores that the underlying processes are frequently underperforming and that a bad professional experience negatively impacts patient outcomes.

95. *Unshackling Innovation* – Health care organizations wanting to reinvent can harness new opportunities by unshackling their smart, innovative team members and outside thinkers to reinvent their organizations for the next 100 years. Those that enable their customers will emerge as the leaders for the next 100 years.

APPENDIX G

WHY DOCTORS ARE RUNNING OUT OF EMPATHY

Those not enmeshed in health care typically are unaware of how dramatically things have changed for physicians. The majority of physicians will no longer recommend their profession to their children. Of course, that is the tip of the iceberg. As mentioned earlier in the book, there are record levels of burnout and even suicide for physicians. The only silver lining is that the experience in far too many hospitals is so appalling for physicians that it leaves many physicians no choice but to either leave the profession or be leaders in the next 100 years of modern medicine. Dr. Mohseni is a good example. He left the toxic work environment and is working on a new health care delivery model to address a large unmet need. The following essay beautifully captures the problems that are far too frequent in hospitals today. As health care is transformed and hospitals either reinvent themselves and their culture or they perish, we shouldn't over-sentimentalize today's hospital environment. It's important that we understand that the underperformance on health outcomes in our status quo health care system is only matched by how much physicians, nurses and other clinicians are frequently victimized in hospitals.

Inside the "sickness-billing industrial complex"

By Alex Mohseni, MD

Walking up to the door of the waiting room, I knew what lay behind it. The gnawing torment would start the day before, or sometimes two days prior. Three parts nausea, two parts dread, and a dash of anxiety — the recipe was always the same. Just add an organic grass-fed doctor, and you have yourself a nice little snack for the healthcare system to chew up and unceremoniously spit out.

This is my story: a successful emergency medicine physician by external parameters, but internally strained. The person who came out of residency — a supremely confident physician ready to take on the world — would never recognize himself 11 years later. My experiences in our healthcare system transformed me, and my story is not unique. There is a sickness that permeates our medical providers within our healthcare system: it is as easy to catch as influenza and as hard to treat.

But before we diagnose this sickness, I would like to describe the context within which we work, this so-called "healthcare system." I find the phrase "healthcare system" difficult to write, because it is an inaccurate representation of what it purports to describe. If we take the word "healthcare" to mean the mishmash of hospitals, doctors, insurance companies, and vendors that profit from our physical and mental maladies, then perhaps it would be more accurate to call it "sickness-billing." It is truly "sickness" rather than "health" that the industry focuses on, and "billing" rather than "care" on which it spends the better portion of its time. And if we take the word "system" to mean an organized set of people working together for a common goal, and if one has ever spent a day in a hospital, then one recognizes that the word "ataxia" better communicates the reality of the experience. "Ataxia" is a medical term we use to describe the inability of a person to move their body in a coordinated way.

But "ataxia" may be too obscure, so I'll use the term "industrial complex" — just think of the patients as our industry's widgets.

This sickness-billing industrial complex, or SBIC — our healthcare system's true identity — is an uncoordinated amalgam of special interests profiting from a series of unintended con- sequences of poorly designed policies. So how did we go from "healthcare" to the SBIC? What happened in the last 20 to 30 years? Here is my version of the story.

Government food policies, such as the subsidization of corn and the promotion of sugar- and carbohydrate-rich foods as "low-fat" alternatives, resulted in a massive increase in calorie-dense, nutrient-poor, and highly processed "foods" in our diet (corn syrup, other sugars, refined wheat, etc.). In addition, societal expectations of portion size and taste transformed as well. These dietary changes have led to dramatic increases in obesity, diabetes, heart disease, cancer, and rates in the United States. The costs borne by Medicare and insurance companies consequently swelled, producing a strained "system" unprepared to handle the increasing need for preventive care. In response to rapidly rising costs, Medicare (to which most insurance companies look for guidance) created a growing number of obstacles to reimbursing doctors and hospitals, and all payers followed suit. These obstacles started as documentation-focused rules, requiring doctors to record a certain number of data points for each medical visit, otherwise reducing reimbursement. This is why your doctor, during your visit for an ankle sprain, may ask if you have had any constipation, vaginal bleeding, or ringing in your ears.

Doctors — often slow, but never dumb — adapted to the new rules, and learned how to recover their lost revenue by spending extra time asking unnecessary questions and documenting endless nonsense in patients' medical charts. Medicare created a game and the doctors learned how to play it, to the detriment of patients. Eventually Medicare piled on even more barriers, which they termed Core Measures. Of course, Medicare couldn't call these things "barriers to paying doctors and hospitals," so it spun the changes as a switch to "value-based care." The problem was, most of the parameters on which it was basing "value" were questionable, with little basis in the scientific literature. Most doctors saw the parameters for what they were: barriers to reimbursement.

Sure enough, the Core Measure program went awry and led to a variety of unintended consequences. At a particular hospital emergency room where I worked, it was decided that all patients who had the remotest possibility of having pneumonia upon their initial evaluation in triage were to be given a dose of antibiotics by mouth immediately, because Medicare had decided that getting antibiotics within six hours of arrival to the ER was a measure of quality. Some patients ended up getting antibiotics they did not need, while others needed IV antibiotics but had just received oral instead. In order to meet our "quality" goal, we were practicing bad medicine.

After doctors and hospitals mastered the Core Measure game, Medicare created yet more games, represented by a seemingly never-ending litany of acronyms that read like a Sesame Street song, from "PQRS," to "MIPS," to "MACRA." These new programs were of such complexity that many doc- tors were faced with three stark choices: 1) spend hundreds of hours trying to learn and adapt to the new rules, 2) sell their practice to a hospital or much larger group (an entity with the resources to hire a consultant to help them figure out how to play the game), or 3) give up and just accept the significantly lower payment.

Sadly, many physicians have opted to sell their practices and give up their autonomy to a corporate entity. This is a major loss to our communities, as independent physician practices are some of the last refuges against the corporate practice of medicine. Just as sad are those doctors who try to stay afloat in the sea of acronyms, barely keeping their heads above water and seeing patients ever more hastily, with less patient face-to-face time, more stress, more rushing, more mistakes, and more frustration — all of which may lead to a dangerous decrease in the physician's capacity for empathy.

None of these new Medicare programs will work to solve the problems within our sickness-billing industrial complex, because we are not dealing with the core fundamental issues: we're treating sickness instead of fostering health, we focus on billing instead of care, and we are completely ataxic (unco- ordinated). We have a very unhealthy population gorging themselves on sugar-rich foods, developing preventable diseases, like type 2 diabetes, with very expensive complications (kidney fail- ure, heart attack, stroke, blindness, etc.), and clinging to unrealistic expectations that doctors and medicines can work miracles to reverse the impact of years of horrendous nutrition. Meanwhile, we have doctors being coerced to spend a majority of their time figuring out how to play documentation games instead of engaging patients in real health-oriented change.

In 2006, within this context of the SBIC, came a fresh, young, eager new emergency medicine doctor. I truly loved learning about and practicing medicine when I began my career. It was exhilarating — the tight-knit teams of nurses, techs, secretaries, physician assistants, and doctors dealing with the chaos of endless streams of patients, with time pressure, challenging problem-solving, and quick decision-making. Great teamwork, amazing saves, and warm appreciation from patients were the norm. Then, in my second year, came my first lawsuit as an attending ("attending" refers to doctors working without supervision, having graduated from residency). It was a case I remembered with photographic precision, because it was one of my most intense. A patient who'd been seen by several previous physicians was admitted for a complaint with a very atypical presentation. The patient later crashed during my shift and my team and I did our best to save him. I remember having a very heartfelt, warm, and sad moment with his family at his bedside before we sent him via helicopter for an emergency surgery that we could not perform at our hospital. Unfortunately, he did not survive. That night, although very saddened about this gentleman's death, I was proud of my team's effort. In court I recounted the scene of the woman from the blood bank running her fastest into the ER with several units of O-negative blood in her hand, knowing that every second counted; every single person was doing everything he or she could to save this man's life.

I felt like a leader of heroes. Yet, we were sued, and treated like criminals. To be sued when you've done something egregiously wrong is understandable. But when you're proud of your own and your team's effort, skill, and decision-making, and cannot imagine what you could have done better, being sued is demoralizing and discombobulating. To be sued when you remember standing by the patient's bedside, your own eyes welling up with tears, because you are a human being who feels the suffering of those around you...

"I did my best. I did what I thought was right. Every medical decision and intervention I made was correct. And somebody hates me so much, they want to ruin my life and end my career. Somebody thinks I did everything wrong. Somebody thinks I am evil." Such was the narrative swimming in my mind for the two years this case was active. Sleepless nights. Stressful shifts. Two years of self-doubt chipping away at my confidence and pride.

When self-doubt takes a foothold in an emergency medicine physician, it is poison. The hallmark of a great ER physician is the confidence to make quick decisions with limited time, information, and resources. No amount of training or knowledge can supplant low confidence, and patients can sense it immediately.

I remember as a young attending I could sense decreasing confidence in some of the older attendings with whom I worked. They shied away from some of the more complicated cases, and we younger attendings would happily take these more challenging cases. I remember thinking to myself back then, "I hope I never lose my confidence." And yet here I was, starting to feel it — and I couldn't understand why.

To my colleagues and bosses, my performance was great. I was seeing patients quickly, providing great medical care, and achieving high patient-satisfaction results. I posted some of the best numbers in my practice for quite a few years, but I felt increasingly unsure of myself. In fact, one of my older colleagues joked to me privately that emergency medicine is the only pro-fession in which you can become more unsure the more you practice it. Not only do ER physicians rank amongst the highest lawsuit rates of all specialties, but they also deal with the unintended complications of medical procedures from every other specialty. This means that the more an emergency medicine doctor practices, the more acutely she experiences all the different tragic ways the SBIC can fail. We learn quickly, from seeing tens of thousands of cases of our own and our colleagues, that no matter how good a doctor you are, you are going to miss certain things, you are going to make mistakes, and certain things are going to happen to your patients that nobody could predict or prevent.

But we also learn that society is not okay with that. Society wants somebody to blame. Family members want somebody to blame. Hospitals want somebody to blame. Society expects perfection. Doctors aren't supposed to make mistakes. I told my colleagues that being a doctor is like being a wildebeest crossing the Mara River: eventually the crocodile is going to snatch one of us and eat him. And then he'll get another, and another, whenever he so chooses, each and every time a devastating shock to the chosen wildebeest and those around him.

In the ensuing few years I saw some of my colleagues get taken down by crocodile lawsuits while I continued to deal with my own. All the while, Medicare ramped up its "value-based" programs, increasing the documentation burden on physicians and hospitals. During the same period, the first and second generations of electronic medical records (EMR) systems were deployed in hospitals. Although intended to streamline medical documentation, EMRs dramatically reduced physician productivity. This was primarily because the EMR companies got away with designing software with horrendous user interfaces and user workflows. How? Unlike most consumer software, in the sickness-billing world those responsible for purchasing software (the hospital C-suite) are not its end users (the medical staff). The EMR developers sold the C-suite on "integration," but nobody paid any attention to usability.

And the cost of these systems is astronomical. In May 2018, the Mayo Clinic announced that they were paying $1.5 billion to switch to the Epic EMR system. Pause for a moment: how could software cost $1.5 billion? Well, when your user interface is so unintuitive that you have to hire and deploy an army of consultants and trainers to hold each user's hand for two weeks, it can lead to truly "epic" implementation costs. As if this were not bad enough, the internet buzzed with stories of Epic bullying anybody who criticized its software. Can you imagine the backlash if Microsoft or Google tried to place gag orders to prevent criticism of their software? Yet this is the world of the SBIC. The negative effects of poorly designed EMRs on physician morale and productivity are well documented.

With reimbursement declining due to Medicare's new rules and doctors becoming less productive because of EMRs, physician practices were forced to make their doctors work faster and leaner than ever before.

My experience as a doctor transformed dramatically as a result of all of these changes. With reimbursement going down due to Medicare's new rules and doctors becoming less productive because of EMRs, physician practices expected their doctors to work faster and leaner than ever before. Hospitals expected increasingly higher patient-satisfaction results. Patients and families expected perfection in care and no complications or unexpected events. Insurance companies expected perfectly documented charts, or else no payment. And EMR vendors expected you to use their dreadful software and keep your mouth shut.

These, then, were our directives: Work faster, make everybody happier, document more, and, oh yeah, don't ever make a mistake.

For myself and many of my colleagues, our mindset before beginning an ER shift flipped from eagerness and energetic anticipation to nausea and dread. One of my colleagues developed this dread of ER shifts before even graduating from residency, and promptly quit emergency medicine the day he graduated. Only later did I truly appreciate what he must have felt.

All physicians and nurses, and especially those in our nation's ERs, make personal sacrifices to enter a profession that provides the opportunity and the honor to heal, comfort, and advise their fellow human beings at all hours of the day. They work weekends, overnights, and holidays while most people are sleeping or spending quality time with friends and family. However, when the constituent forces in the SBIC described above repeatedly insult and interfere with the humanity and virtue of medical providers, they do great damage to the provider's ability to empathize.

This loss of empathy is the sickness within our providers to which I referred at the beginning of this essay. Every condition needs a name, so I shall coin the term "empathitis." Empathy, in my personal perspective of its application to the medical profession, is the ability to preserve your sense that you are treating another human being. They're not just "room 12," or "the hypertensive stroke patient," but a human being with a name, a story, family, friends, hopes, and fears — a human being who deserves your full attention, your touch, and your diligent and meticulous thoughtfulness.

Empathitis: an acute or chronic reduction in a person's ability to empathize, often affecting his/her work and life performance. When the forces surrounding me made it difficult for me to be the type of physician I wanted to be and had trained to be, when those forces repeatedly directed my attention to documentation, billing, EMRs, and moving patients as fast as possible, and when those forces continually chipped away at my mountain of empathy, reducing it to scarcely a handful, I knew the time had come to say goodbye to emergency medicine. My last ER shift was in the summer of 2017.

Luckily, my departure did not signify the end of my medical career. I was fortunate to have worked for a medical practice that gave me the opportunity to develop skills and experience in healthcare technology, data analytics, business development, and telemedicine, and now I have the great pleasure of practicing telemedicine with CirrusMD, an innovative group of amazing human beings who are transforming how healthcare is delivered. Now, when I see patients from my computer screen, I can chat with them as long as I want. They share stories with me and sometimes we laugh. I advise them the same as I would advise my own family. We don't rush anything. More often than not, they just need reassurance and a little bit of guidance. Although I am no longer placing central lines or doing intubations, I feel more like a true physician than ever before. I spend time talking to patients about health and not just sickness. In addition to dealing with whatever the patient's acute medical condition might be, we talk about food choices, exercise regimens, sleeping habits, behavior modifications, and stress-reduction techniques, and how these things may be connected to the patient's acute condition. Sometimes we discuss fears and anxieties; I've even coached patients through full-blown panic attacks. Now I can truly focus on health and care, not just sickness and billing. Now I operate in a system that I actually like to use and supports me and my mission.

I feel blessed, but I know that many of my former colleagues and friends in the world of emergency medicine continue to endure and suffer. Less than half of my residency class is still practicing traditional emergency medicine. In an era of doctor shortages and long wait times in ERs, I felt this story was important to share, so that you might have some sense as to what lies behind the waiting room door.

Alex Mohseni is a physician innovator and problem solver who is deeply interested in building systems to solve health care's many challenges.

APPENDIX H

DECODING A FULLY-INSURED RENEWAL (MICHIGAN)

A health insurance renewal is not as complicated as it seems. Although you may be unfamiliar with the terminology, each section and calculation is intended to predict a premium that (when paid) will fund the following:

1. Upcoming 12 months medical & Rx claims (what we want paid)
2. Stop-Loss premiums to reduce exposure to high cost claimants (negotiable)
3. Carrier's operating expenses & profit (negotiable)

The following is an actual de-identified 2018 renewal; yours will look the same:

Renewal Development - Detailed Projections

	Medical	Prescription Drug	Dental	Vision	Total
Average Monthly Employees Enrolled in Experience Period	163	163			163
Average Monthly Members Enrolled in Experience Period	341	341			341
1. Approved Charges	$1,819,597	$531,207			$2,350,804
Less: Provider Reimbursement Savings	$887,609	$264,249			$1,151,858
Less: Member Liability	$248,556	$37,710			$286,266
2. Claims Paid in Experience Period	$683,432	$228,880			$912,312
Less Large Claim Payment	$130,253	$3,216			$133,469
3. Net Claims Considered for Rating Projection	$553,179	$225,664			$778,843
Plus: Estimated Incurred But Not Reported Claims	$32,648	$384			$33,032
4. Total Incurred Claims	$585,827	$226,048			$811,875
Annualized Incurred Claims	$585,827	$226,048			$811,875
5. Adjustment for Membership and Benefit Changes during the experience period	$49,316	($8,350)			$40,966
Annualized Incurred Claims adjusted for benefit and membership changes	$635,143	$217,698			$852,840
Effective Trend	1.0818	1.1965			1.1111
6. Trended Claims	$687,111	$260,484			$947,595
Plus: Estimated Provider Adjustment	$48,892	($44,543)			$4,350
Plus: Large Claims up to Attachment Point	$97,591	$2,409			$100,000
Plus: Capitation	$62,527	$0			$62,527
Plus: Adjustment for Credibility	($30,735)	$568			($30,167)
7. Projected Claims for the Rating Period	$865,386	$218,919			$1,084,305
Plus: Pooling Charges	$146,756	$24,790			$171,548
Plus: Projected Retention Expenses	$256,268	$29,876			$286,144
Less: Cap/Floor Adjustment	$0	$0			$0
8. Projected Total Expenses for the Rating Period	$1,268,413	$273,585			$1,541,998
9. Projected Income Required for the Rating Period	$1,268,413	$273,585			$1,541,998
10. Annual Income at Current Rates	$1,123,983	$241,059			$1,365,043
11. Change in Rates for the Rating Period expressed as a Percentage Change from your Current Rates	12.85%	13.49%			12.96%

- Some variances may occur due to rounding.

Experience Period: (Incurred: 08/2016-07/2017), (Paid: 08/2016-08/2017)

Here's how it looks when we categorize into the three "buckets":

Renewal Development - Detailed Projections

	Medical	Prescription Drug	Dental	Vision	Total
Average Monthly Employees Enrolled in Experience Period	163	163			163
Average Monthly Members Enrolled in Experience Period	341	341			341
1. Approved Charges	$1,819,597	$531,207			$2,350,804
Less: Provider Reimbursement Savings	$887,609	$264,249			$1,151,858
Less: Member Liability	$248,556	$37,710			$286,266
2. Claims Paid in Experience Period	$683,432	$228,880			$912,312
Less Large Claim Payment	$130,253	$3,216			$133,469
3. Net Claims Considered for Rating Projection	$553,179	$225,664			$778,843
Plus: Estimated Incurred But Not Reported Claims	$32,648	$384			$33,032
4. Total Incurred Claims	$585,827	$226,048			$811,875
Annualized Incurred Claims	$585,827	$226,048			$811,875
5. Adjustment for Membership and Benefit Changes during the experience period	$49,316	($8,350)			$40,966
Annualized Incurred Claims adjusted for benefit and membership changes	$635,143	$217,698			$852,840
Effective Trend	1.0818	1.1965			1.1111
6. Trended Claims	$687,111	$260,484			$947,595
Plus: Estimated Provider Adjustment	$48,892	($44,543)			$4,350
Plus: Large Claims up to Attachment Point	$97,591	$2,409			$100,000
Plus: Capitation	$62,527	$0			$62,527
Plus: Adjustment for Credibility	($30,735)	$568			($30,167)
7. Projected Claims for the Rating Period	$865,386	$218,919			$1,084,305
Plus: Pooling Charges	$146,756	$24,790			$171,548
Plus: Projected Retention Expenses	$256,268	$29,876			$286,144
Less: Cap/Floor Adjustment	$0	$0			$0
8. Projected Total Expenses for the Rating Period	$1,268,413	$273,585			$1,541,998
9. Projected Income Required for the Rating Period	$1,268,413	$273,585			$1,541,998
10. Annual Income at Current Rates	$1,123,983	$241,059			$1,365,043
11. Change in Rates for the Rating Period expressed as a Percentage Change from your Current Rates	12.85%	13.49%			12.96%

Annotations:

Claims - Medical & Rx
$1,270,668 Total Claims
- $286,266 Members
$984,402 Claims Paid

Stop Loss Insurance
$171,548
($33,469) Paid over spec
$138,079 Profit

Operations & Profit
$94,750 Trend
$4,350 Provider Adj
$286,144 Retention
($30,167) Credibility
$138,079 Stop Loss Profit
$493,156 (50% claims)
$3,025 PEPY
$252.12 PEPM

- Some variances may occur due to rounding.

Experience Period: (Incurred: 08/2016-07/2017), (Paid: 08/2016-08/2017)

Each "bucket" explained:

1. Upcoming 12 months medical & Rx claims

The important facts to consider are included below. I have omitted "Provider Reimbursement Savings" as this is the carrier's way of marketing a discount that is superficial at best. This discount is the amount the carrier purportedly negotiates from the Approved Charges submitted by providers. The Approved Charges come from the provider/hospital Charge Master, which is grossly inflated to account for the agreed discount. *We need to focus on what is actually paid. Here's how to add it all up:*

Net Claims Considered for Rating Projection $778,843

This number is derived by taking Approved Charges, deducting discounts (above), member liability (deductibles, coinsurance, & copays), and removing "high claimant" charges. This is where we start.

Add: IBNR (Incurred but not received) $33,032

IBNR is a legitimate consideration due to claim billing lag. However, this amount only represents an estimate.

Add: Large Claims Up to Attachment Point $100,000

Although this is in the "Trended Claims" section of the report, include this in your total claim calculations. In this example it is $100,000, which represents the amount paid for a high claimant. Yes, it looks like self-insuring and it is, in a way. The difference is that you pay for it about one year after it is incurred (at your renewal). So, in this example, the group had only one employee exceed the "pooling point" or "attachment point." Thus, $100,000 is added back. We'll discuss this further in Stop-Loss below.

Add: Capitation $62,527

This may be a new term for you, but it's actually pretty simple. Instead of the carrier paying primary care providers per visit, they pay selected in-network PCPs a fixed monthly amount for each of your members who nominate a "capitated provider." This amount is paid whether or not your employee goes to the doctor. If your employee does not have a regular doctor, a capitated provider is assigned. In this case, it equates to $183.36 per member (including spouses and children). This pays for about two visits per year. You may pay more for capitation, and I believe it discourages quality care. Here are a few important questions to consider:

1. Do you think every member goes to the PCP two times a year?
2. If the PCP cannot bill insurance for your visit, are they motivated to spend time with you?
3. If you're on an HSA plan, does the member still pay for the visit, even if your PCP is "capitated?"
4. Is the HMO network restrictive enough to steer patients to low cost, high quality providers?

TOTAL Claims Paid: $984,402 [not listed]

This amount is not specifically listed on the renewal example above. However, it is the most important statistic you need to calculate (see the green bubble). It includes all Medical & Rx incurred for a 12-month period.

2. *Stop-Loss premiums to reduce exposure to high cost claimants*

You may be aware of the reinsurance market if you've ever considered self-funding. Primarily known as stop-loss insurance, it is purchased by fully-insured carriers and self-funded employers alike.

Pooling Charges: $171,546

This amount is the cost of stop-loss insurance for severe, high cost claims. It is the premium you pay for the insurance company to accept this risk. In this example, your responsibility is the first $100,000 of a big claim. Called the "attachment point" or pooling point, payments in excess of $100,000 per member, are excluded from your claim experience & premium calculation. (NOTE: I've seen this credit conveniently omitted, make sure you see it in writing). The $100,000 deductible includes medical and Rx payments combined, per member. So, if you have 10 members exceed $100,000, your renewal will reflect a $1,000,000 increase, plus everything else!

Less: Large Claim Payments: $133,469, but really only $33,469....

In section 2 [Less large claims payments], you see $133,469 was removed from "Claims Paid in Experience Period" (This is the credit you're looking for). This means that the entire group of large claimants had a total of $133,469 in claims paid. In section 6 [Large Claim Payments up to Attachment Point] you see $100,000 added back to your premium calculation. This tells you two things; there was only one large claimant, and the stop-loss insurance paid a net $33,469 after receiving $171,546 in premium.

One question to ask as we review each of these "buckets" is: if my group maintains historical medical utilization, who keeps the proceeds from each bucket? When you're negotiating a fully-insured renewal, every dollar increase is spread over your monthly single/double/family rate for the next 12 months.

3. Carrier's operating expenses & profit.

Adjustment for Membership & Benefit Changes, ADD: $40,966

Adjustments will be applied for group demographic changes. Demographic changes include high turnover, mid-year open enrollment that changes member responsibility, or a group wide benefit change. In this example, the group chose to add a 5th tier to the Rx card, resulting in a higher copay for members taking specialty drugs. This should reduce premium. However, high turnover is also present in this group. Ask for clarity on what changed and why any adjustments were made that increased the premium.

Effective Trend: 1.1111 or ADD: $94,755.

Actuarially, trend is the year-over-year % increase in claims expense. Practically, it is a function that insurance companies and health care providers use to automatically increase revenue. Trend is a historical look back that is then projected forward. This creates a self-fulfilling prophecy, resulting in an auto-increase for both your insurance company, and the health care providers they pay. It has been accepted as norm for years. Fight the urge to accept this as fact.

Previously, I mentioned if you're considering self-funding, you should apply a "trend" factor to your Expected Claims budget. I only recommend this if you have poor claims data. It's your money to budget and if trend is less than expected, you win. Good carriers have nearly perfect claims data, and projected claims in excess of your current claims period should only be justified by knowledge of an ongoing/new high claimant(s).

Don't let carriers automatically apply trend to your premium. Instead, ask them to provide the last two year's contract with the hospitals in your area showing the charge master and discount per CPT code. Also, ask for your PBM's (prescription benefit manager) prescription contract with retail cost of each drug and the carrier's own discounted rate. If trend is in excess of Consumer Price Index (CPI normally about 2%), ask why the cost was allowed to increase.

Estimated Provider Adjustments, ADD: $4,350

This is, again, a fairly opaque adjustment. When I asked what this adjustment includes, here is the response from the carrier:

"Benefit expense items that do not run through our claims process-ing systems. These items include payments to providers for risk arrangements, hospital settlements, provider incentives and phar-macy rebates."

If we break that down, essentially, it's a bucket of adjust-ments for paying or receiving money outside of contract. For example, drug manufacturers provide rebates as a result of PBM negotiation. Depending on your PBM, you receive 0-100% of these rebates as credit towards your renewal. In our example, one can assume that the carrier received $44,543 in Rx rebates.

However, this was "washed out" by $48,892 in risk arrange-ments, hospital settlements, or provider incentives. Ask for details on these expenses that apply directly to your group.

Specifically, get the list of Rx rebates received showing total rebate, carrier retention, and your credit. As for risk arrange-ments and hospital settlements, if it doesn't apply directly to your group, ask for it to be removed.

ADD: Projected Retention Expense, ADD: $286,144

This is a clever way to say "markup." Here is the carrier's actual definition:

"The amount charged to customers to cover the costs of pro-viding services. This includes: claim processing, customer ser-vice, wellness and care management, access to carrier negotiated provider discounts and data and analytics (reporting)."

Don't get me wrong, markup is necessary to cover opera-tions, G&A, overhead, and profit. Without markup, we cannot operate. So, the best way to analyze this line item is to benchmark against industry peers. In this example, the $286,144 represents this carrier's markup. However, to make this number meaning-ful, we need to change it to a PEPM (per employee per month) cost. This group has 163 enrolled, so the PEPM is $146.29, with a member/employee ratio of 2.09.

Below are some recent industry-peer mark-ups. I've included claim processing, customer service, wellness & care management, network negotiation fees, claims reporting, and agent commission in each of these benchmarks:

-Carrier #1: $146.29 PEPM (fully-insured) & $96.65 PEPM (self-funded)

-Carrier #2: $85.55 PEPM (fully-insured) & $78.56 PEPM (self-funded)

-Carrier #3: $69.10 PEPM (self-funded)

-Carrier #4: $52.49 PEPM + hourly case management (self-funded)

-Clearly, Carrier #1 is nearly 3x the lowest competitor in the market, and represents the highest markup.

Accordingly, one would expect a significant benefit for this markup. To validate this, ask the following simple questions:

-Are you receiving claims processing worth 200%-300% of market?

-Are you receiving customer service worth 200-300% of market?

-Are you receiving wellness & care management worth 200-300% of market?

-If I'm paying 11% trend, is the network negotiation worth 200-300% of market?

-Is claims transparency, analytics, and plan counseling worth 200-300% of market?

-Is my agent/advisor receiving 200-300% of market commission to service my account?

CONCLUSION

Hopefully, this helps sheds light on the way an insurance carrier calculates a renewal premium, so you have leverage at the negotiating table. In this example, $493,156 (50% markup on claims) could flow through to the insurance carrier.

That's $3,025 per enrolled employee per year! What would that mean to your bottom line and/or employees' wallet?

BENEFITS OPTIONS FOR SMALL BUSINESSES AND SOLE PROPRIETORS

By David Contorno

I am a small business (or individual)... how can I create a benefits package in the Health Rosetta mindset?

Health Rosetta is more a mindset than a single strategy, a collection of principles and practices rather than a health plan. While there are some regulatory and market conditions that make it easier to follow this model as an employer group gets larger, there are still some things that anyone can do.

Small Businesses

Within the ACA, a small employer was defined as one with fewer than 100 full time equivalent employees (FTEs). However, in October 2015, President Obama signed the PACE act allowing each state to decide to either keep its traditional definition (50 employees in most cases) or go to 100. Most states opted to keep it at 50, although some states, NY for example, moved it or kept it at 100. So, from a regulatory perspective, 50 employees or fewer seems to be the most common "small group." As an employer moves up in size, some of the financing side strategies definitely become easier.

Although all of our strategies are common sense, they are still innovative to health care, and small businesses do have to get even more "non-traditional" to accomplish similar results. The primary reason is that the ACA put more restrictions on the products insurance carriers can offer in this space; in addition, there is the possibility that larger-sized small employers may be subject to certain ACA mandates that these plans may not comply with.

Mandates, however, do not apply to most employers under 50 FTEs. This means there is no penalty for offering non-ACA compliant plans (or even no coverage). For this size employer, there are a few potential solutions:

1. Contract with a local direct primary care (DPC) doctor for your employees. Studies show that for about 80 percent of people, a proper functioning primary care home can provide 100 percent of the care they need. The national average cost is $50-$150 per employee per month. There are generally no additional fees, no co-pays, and no claims to file.

2. Primary care alone cannot serve the needs of the remaining 20 percent and can leave other people anxious about the "what if's". In this case, a "health sharing plan" can provide that additional protection. While many of these plans came out of a faith-based exemption under the ACA, several have developed in recent years that either remove or significantly downplay the religious affiliation requirements. Ironically, although most sharing organizations want to avoid any traditional insurance terms, for fear of being regulated like insurance, most operate the way insurance was always intended to operate: All members pay enough into the pot to fund judicious and fair disbursements of benefits to cover moderate to large medical encounters. (The small to moderate stuff should either be paid for out of pocket or handled by the DPC

doctor mentioned in #1 above.) A good sharing program will recognize the benefits of DPC and give a discount on the membership fees when included. I priced out a family of four, with DPC and the sharing program (with an initial patient responsibility of $1000 per medical need) in Western North Carolina and the total cost for all was well under $700 per month for the whole family. I have seen many single premiums in traditional programs at this price point lately.

3. If DPC is not an option, either because you have a highly distributed workforce or because there simply aren't any near you, you may still be able to bring in many of its benefits of primary care in a virtual format. Generally, this costs around $100 per month for an employee.

4. Lastly, as the Association Health Plan (AHP) Rule rolls out, it *may* offer an opportunity for employers to more easily band together. Contrary to widespread misconceptions, I believe this will only give such groups access to limited benefits. However, it could lift small businesses out of the small group market, which operates under community rating requirements. If so, this would allow a Health Rosetta advisor to construct a plan that truly addresses incentives designed to reward quantity over quality in ways not otherwise available to smaller groups.

Larger Small Businesses

As an employer moves out of the 50-employee market, regulations become more onerous, but at the same time, it becomes easier to operate in a Health Rosetta environment. Here are a few points to consider for employers of 50 to about 100:

1. Contrary to popular belief, self-insured does not inherently mean more risky; it can actually be less risky than a fully insured plan if you want it to be. Risk can be the result of an inexperienced benefits broker but it can also be

a deliberate choice. Due to the pressure the ACA applied to fully insured plans, there are today many new forms of protection or risk management for smaller employers, e.g., aggregate-only policies, spaggregate, monthly aggregate accommodation, non-laserable contracts, and, as mentioned in #2, level funding (not to be confused with carrier-based level funding).

2. Not all self-inured plans are created equal. If you take a fully insured large carrier plan, and put that same plan, PPO network, pharmacy benefit management, etc., into a self-insured model, you have functionally changed absolutely nothing. You still have relinquished full control of both costs and utilization to an entity that benefits as costs rise. Also, most carriers expressly prohibit Health Rosetta principles because they actively lower costs—which in turn lowers their profit.

3. A "level funded plan" is often viewed as a safe, "dip a toe in the water" path to becoming self-insured. When the carriers saw this happening, they came out with their own versions and designed them to maximize profit. They do this by inflating the fixed costs, reducing the claims funding, and, in the rare case where there is leftover claims funding, keeping one-third to one-half of what you overpaid. With a proper level-funded model, the self-insured employer gets far more control, far more flexibility, reduced fixed costs, and 100 percent of the excess claims funding back.

4. Once an employer determines that it can construct a financially feasible self-insured arrangement with a proper third-party administrator and PBM, all the Health Rosetta principles can easily be applied.

5. These plans can and should be designed to meet all the ACA mandates for both the employer and the individual.

Individuals

What can you do as an employee not in a decision-making capacity at a company, or as someone who is self-employed or unemployed? You can do a lot! First off, please remember that health insurance does *not* equal health care. Health insurance is just one way to pay for care. Another is the health sharing programs mentioned above, which have been operating for a couple of decades and are used by approximately one million people. And there is still another way: It's called cash.

The tens of millions of people with high deductible plans can save enormous sums by using cash, as demonstrated by my own hernia operation. Even using a facility 800 miles away from my home, which had much higher quality than any in my area, and paying 100 percent of my own costs, including travel, I paid one-third of what my out-of-pocket would have been had I stayed local and used a traditional insurance plan. Most of the time, you do not need to travel anywhere near that far to find a high-quality facility, but if you were going to get way better care and save thousands of dollars, wouldn't you be willing to?

These same principles can be applied to prescriptions. Especially with generics, the cash price is often below your plan's co-pay. And when you unknowingly overpay for the drug by showing your insurance ID card, you are actually hurting yourself down the road in the form of higher premiums—and you are often hurting the pharmacy thanks to "clawbacks." This is when your plan's PBM pulls back the difference between the co-pay and cost of the drug in order to enhance their profits, even though they literally provided no value, especially in that particular transaction.

It may not be easy, because the system doesn't want it to be, but for an individual, the solution is relatively simple: You need to demand total cost and quality information (getting that is the hard part), compare these data with your insurance coverage, and only then decide where to go for care. Instead, most Americans take an "insurance first" approach. In nearly all other economic transactions, we determine best value first, then we figure out how to get the money needed to pay for it. If we all did that in health care, things would change for the positive *very* rapidly.

Appendix

CASE STUDIES

This chapter highlights wise employers and smart benefit strategies that have created replicable microcosms of high-per- forming health care systems as good as any in the world. It's in employers' enlightened self-interest to follow suit.

CASE STUDY:

Copper State Bolt & Nut Company

Advisor Organization:	Wincline
Headquarters:	Phoenix, AZ
Industry:	Manufacturing
Sector:	Private
Client Size:	500+ Employees
Employees On Plan:	313
Total Lives On Plan	586
Plan funding:	Self-funded
Case Study:	1/1/2017 - 12/31/2019

Key Takeaways

1. Reduced health care spending from $500+ (PEPM) in 2017 to under $300 (PEPM) in 2019.
2. Achieved a 40% savings in just two years. Over $1.3 million annually
3. Employee's pay $0 (deductible waived) when seeking second opinion

Testimonial

"Without Wincline's involvement, I have no doubt that an employee would have unnecessarily had his colon removed if the plan did not require a qualified second opinion. This saved the employee from unnecessary life-changing surgery and improved the quality of his life. Instead, he received another recommended surgery all for 9% of what would have been paid in years past saving the employee and plan hundreds of thousands of dollars. Now, Copper State gets a capable, loyal and productive employee who appreciates what was done for him."

Sam Tiffany, Human Resources Manager,
Copper State Bolt & Nut Co.

"What I like about Wincline is their commitment to end the dirty data, provide complete transparency, and the belief they can transform health care."

Sarah Shannon, President,
Copper State Bolt & Nut Co.

Client Background

Copper State Nut & Bolt was combating rising health care costs on a carrier-based partially self-funded plan. Previously they didn't have any strategy to handle the rising health care costs and were simply reacting and accepting the renewal rate increases year after year. In 2017, Copper State Nut & Bolt was facing a 30% rate increase from their incumbent carrier when Health Rosetta Advisor John Harvey, and his firm Wincline, took over. To combat rising costs it had three main goals: 1) cut unnecessary health care costs, 2) reduce employee cost, and 3) reduce unnecessary waste and misaligned incentives in the plan.

Copper State Nut & Bolt is a manufacturer based out of Phoenix, AZ with over 30 locations across the US. They are a specialty manufacturer that provides an array of products to the industrial, manufacturing and construction industries. Prior to changing plans, Copper State was overspending on health care while the old-line carrier was unnecessarily profiting from Copper State's health plan through misaligned incentives and excessive hidden fees.

Advisor Background

John founded Wincline in June 2016 with over a decade of experience in sales and the employee benefits industry. He did so with a simple mission: To change the way employers experience health care by eliminating the greed and inefficiency in the benefits industry.

As a fee-only, independent employee benefits advisor, John specializes in working with his clients to navigate cost-saving, higher quality benefit solutions. He strives to first understand the company's business, and only then designs innovative benefits plans to align with their corporate objectives.

John leads his team with a broad base of specialties including employee communications, benefits technology, plan design analysis, and consumer-driven health plans. He's been in this industry long enough to know what works and what doesn't. As such, he's highly effective at cutting through the nonsense and uncovering waste, fraud, and mismanagement in the health care industry.

Approach

Copper State Bolt & Nut was continuing to face year over year of rising health care costs without a strategy to manage their health plan. In 2017, Copper State Bolt & Nut partnered with Wincline, a fee only advisory firm that aligned with their interests, to create a proactive healthcare strategy to reduce costs, remove excess waste in the plan and improve overall benefits for the employees.

Through active plan management and aligned interests, Copper State Bolt & Nut was able to identify that their existing partially self-funded plan was being mismanaged and root out waste that was increasing the profits of the carrier. John Harvey helped Copper State Bolt & Nut by guiding them through a two-year process moving off a Cigna self-funded bundled plan an onto a transparent open-network approach leveraging reference based reimbursement and direct contracts.

This transition to Copper State Bolt & Nut reducing year over year costs and gaining control of their health care expenses did not come without its surprises and challenges. First, in 2017 Wincline helped Copper State Bolt & Nut transition from a paid stop-loss contract to an incurred stop-loss contract providing the necessary risk management to protect the plan and it's employees. In addition, Wincline identified nearly $100k in outstanding stop-loss reimbursements that the old carrier failed to issue back to the plan.

Further investigation found that the incumbent plan was paying a large portion of carrier fees through claims portion of the medical plan, which is often how carriers include hidden and unscrutinized fees. One of these fees was a "Medical Shared Savings Fee" that charged Copper State Bolt & Nut 3% (not to exceed $3,000 per claim) of the provider's billed charges for each individual in-network claim. Putting administrative fees inside the medical plan and claims reimbursement is a practice that carriers leverage to reduce their fixed administrative fees in order to appear competitive with other carriers. Wincline was able to advise Copper State Bolt & Nut by identifying and separating all the fixed fees from the medical plan so that Copper State Bolt & Nut had a clearer picture of the excessive administrative fees.

Also, Copper State Bolt & Nut discovered that it's old carrier-administrator was applying their use of in-network benefits to out-of-network providers to increase their "cost containment fees" but were not administering the plan correctly as they were outlined in the plan documents. Copper State Bolt & Nut plan documents expressed clearly that there were no out-of network benefits on the plan. However the old carrier was using their network adequacy program that gave them authorization to use in-network benefits to out-of-network providers that boosted the carrier's own so-called "cost containment" fees.

In addition, after identifying waste, hidden fees and blatant mismanagement, Wincline helped Copper State Bolt & Nut partner with an independent TPA, execute an independent stop-loss contract, and leverage a transparent open network with reference based reimbursement to reduce the overall health plan costs. This approach was the main driver Copper State Bolt & Nut leveraged to reduce its health care spending by 40%, or $1.3 million annually, compared to their incumbent carrier plan.

To help plan members and employees take advantage of their new health plan, Wincline created the Member Champion role to address employee questions, navigate members and drive members through optimal care pathways (second opinions, primary care, physical therapy, musculoskeletal surgeries, and more). The new member champion position was key to assisting members through the complex health care system to getting optimal high value care. In addition to engaging members and creating a member champion position, Copper State Nut & Bolt required second opinions for surgeries to ensure the member was getting the best care possible. Plus, if a member sought a second opinion and still needed surgery, there would be no cost to the member and deductible would be waived. This made the smart choice the easy choice.

Top-Level Results

Two years after partnering with an independent, fee-only advisor firm, Wincline, helped Copper State Bolt & Nut reduce health plan costs by 40%, a savings of $1.3 million annually.

It's per employee per month (PEPM) went down significantly from $500+ PEPM to under $300 PEPM allowing Copper State Bolt & Nut to reinvest these savings into improving overall employee benefits.

Through active plan management, a new member champion position and smart care pathways, Copper State Bolt & Nut was able to provide superior health care and benefits to its members and completely waive deductibles and all costs for members when pursuing the high-value care pathway. In addition to employees saving money it saved a lot of unnecessary care and improved employees overall experience in their health care journey. The employer is now able to reinvest those savings back into providing better benefits for their employees over the long term.

CASE STUDY:

Gasparilla Inn & Club

Advisor Organization:	Mitigate Partners
Headquarters:	Boca Grande, Florida
Industry:	Service and Hospitality (seasonal)
Sector:	Private
Client Size:	450 total, 270 benefit eligible
Employees On Plan:	130 for 6 months of year / 215 for 6 months = 185 average for the year
Total Lives On Plan	327
Plan funding:	Self-funded
Plan Year:	7/1 - 6/30
Case Study:	7/1/2016 - 6/30/2019

Key Takeaways

1. Reduced health care spending by 34%, saving $1.8 million over 3 years
2. No increases for 4 years
3. Eliminated deductibles, from $2,500 Individual / $4,500 Family to $0

Client Testimonial

"We're saving probably between five and ten thousand dollars a year as a family, that's the difference between a few mortgage payments and college savings for my son"

Nathan McKelvy,
Assistant Food and Beverage Director at Gasparilla Inn

Client Background

Gasparilla Inn & Club is an upscale island resort on the Southwest Gulf Coast of Florida that was suffering from rising health care costs year after year.

From 2013 to 2016, Gasparilla Inn had a 12% average increase per year in health insurance premiums under its fully insured plan with a traditional publicly traded carrier. During this time period Gasparilla Inn was also overspending on health care. On average, its health claims spending was 35% below the amount of premiums collected a year (65% loss ratio), which benefited their carrier's bottomline. Gasparilla Inn's total health care spend with the old plan was projected to increase to $1.3 million in July 2016, threatening the resort's ability to provide benefits to its employees.

To combat rising costs, Gasparilla Inn had three main goals: 1) cut spending, 2) reduce employee cost, and 3) minimize member disruption.

Advisor Background

Carl Schuessler is the managing principal at Mitigate Partners in Atlanta, Georgia. Mitigate Partners is a Risk Management, Cost Containment and Employee Benefits Consulting firm, which is a partnership of fourteen employee benefit consulting and brokerage firms that allows local management within a collaborative environment with more than 330 years of combined experience.

Carl has been working as an insurance, risk management, and employee benefits consultant for over thirty years. His focus is treating the employer's money like his own. Mitigate Partners goal is to provide best-in-class benefits at substantially lower costs, while improving clinical and financial outcomes for employers and health plan members.

He is an advocate of active health care management and saying no to passive, status quo health care plans that reward insurers more than plan sponsors and its members. Carl has helped large and small companies across various industries regain control over their health care benefits by creating innovative health care plans that meet the specific needs of their employees to achieve their financial goals.

Approach

Carl was able to gain the trust of C-level executives by exposing how much its old health plan was draining its finances. He worked directly with the CFO and CEO to create a vision of improved clinical outcomes, coupled with better financial outcomes for the employer and employees.

One of Gasparilla Inn's main goals was to increase health care and health benefits education among its employees. Prior to implementing the new plan on July 1, 2016, Gasparilla Inn conducted six Benefits Education meetings in June 2016 to help employees understand their new benefits before the big change. Gasparilla has continued to hold these meetings annually, every June, to ensure employees remain informed about their health benefits.

In addition to rising health spending Gasparilla Inn had several challenges. The first obstacle had to do with its employees. Due to the nature of its business as a resort, Gasparilla Inn only operates during October to July, so most of its employees are seasonal workers. They have 130 employees on its health care plan for the first six months of the year and then a total of 215 employees on its plan for the second half of the year. On average, Gasparilla Inn has 185 employees on its health care plan year-round.

In January 2016, the Affordable Care Act (ACA) came into effect. This made employee enrollment more challenging as the ACA mandated that all employees who returned in October 2015 and had accumulated the required hours must be offered coverage.

The second challenge was a product of Gasparilla Inn's location. The Southwest Gulf Coast is one of the nation's most expensive regions for health care, with up to 2,000% markups for common treatments and procedures like knee replacements and CT scans. Price variation is a major issue in standard Prefered Provider Organization (PPO) network contracts. Quality scores are equally as important, as there are high quality, low cost providers and low quality, high cost providers. Good plans actively manage the affordability and value of health care options and services.

Cost of CT Scan in Tampa

System (location)	Avg. Billed	Avg. Cost	Medicare Pays	Units of Service
Florida Hospital (Tampa)	$5,193	$ 80	$168	3,545
St. Joseph's (Tampa)	$4,244	$107	$167	6,508
Brandon Reg. (Tampa)	$8,022	$ 67	$166	3,318
Morton Plant (Clearwater)	$4,136	$ 49	$165	5,145
Palms of Pasadena (St. Petersburg)	$7,301	$110	$179	2,166
Sarasota Memorial (Sarasota)	$3,529	$145	$185	15,725

The graph shows average cost, Medicare pricing, and average billed amount for a CT scan across six hospitals in Tampa, Florida. Traditional carrier networks contract a discount off billed charges resulting in exorbitant health care spending for plan sponsors.

Carl was tasked with providing better, more affordable coverage for all employees. In order to find the root cause of the resort's rising health costs, he pulled a report detailing the resort's health care spending from 2013 to 2016, a time period when Gasparilla Inn was still under a traditional fully insured plan. Carl discovered that the resort was overspending on health care, as claims paid were only 65% of the amount of premiums resulting in a huge profit for the carrier.

After exposing this to Gasparilla Inn, Carl worked with its executives and leaders to move the resort off its fully insured plan and construct a better, more affordable health insurance plan.

Top-Level Results

In July 2016, Gasparilla Inn moved off its fully insured plan onto a self-funded plan. By July 2019 it had saved over $1.8 million – a 34% reduction. Under the new plan, Gasparilla Inn is projected to save $5 million over the next five years.

When faced with a decision to go self-funded, Gasparilla Inn considered working with a traditional insurance carrier, but instead chose its current self-funded health plan. In light of what the traditional carrier projections were for 2016 to 2018, the cumulative savings are $3.8 million -- a 67% reduction from what it would have been had they stayed with the old-line carrier.

With Carl's help Gasparilla Inn achieved its first goal of reducing health care costs. Its Per Employee Per Year (PEPY) Medical Expense average is now $2,993 – 75% under the national average – and its Per Member Per Month (PMPM) Prescription Drug Expense average is now $47.53 – 48% under the national average.

Gasparilla Inn's employees don't have copays for any imaging when performed at one of its directly contracted providers. This translates into significant savings for employees, as the average cost of MRIs/CT scans in the Southwest Gulf Coast of Florida can cost well over $1,200, one employee received a claim worth $38,400.

Carl devised a plan that focuses heavily on value-based care, making preventative medicine and procedures like cancer screenings extremely affordable or free. For example, employees can receive a preventative colonoscopy covered at 100%, including polyp removal during the same visit if they are found. Under the

ACA, preventive colonoscopies are covered at 100%, however if polyps are found, the removal is classified as a diagnostic code and billed as a separate charge to the patient. Diagnostic colonoscopies are more expensive than preventative and in the Tampa area the procedure can range from $1,300 to upwards of $19,000.

The new plan also had a direct impact on employees. Gasparilla Inn employees used to pay a $2,500 (single) and $4,500 (family) deductible, which was a lot compared to the average employee salary. Today, they have a $0 deductible with significantly reduced or nonexistent copays.

Gasparilla Inn's new plan eliminated the risk of expensive out-of-network fees and surprise medical billing, as employees now have no network restrictions and are free to go to any hospital or clinician in the U.S.

The new plan focuses on value-based care with an emphasis on increased access to direct primary care services and affordable preventative treatments. Employees now have access to free primary care services, including transportation to appointments if necessary.

Employees were also given more accessible options for primary care, such as a clinic that is 400 yards from the resort. Primary care providers are funded through a value-based care model – not fee-for-service – meaning clinicians are rewarded for improved health outcomes instead of the number of services provided.

Using the significant savings it accrued from changing health plans, Gasparilla Inn hired a Benefits Champion, Liz Schrock, in July 2016. Liz is responsible for the administration of all aspects of the employee benefits program. Her main role is to educate more than 215 employees year-round about their health benefits and how to make smart health care decisions. Gasparilla Inn employees have the ability to go to Liz for any health care benefits questions. She also works with community partners to resolve complex claims. She is considered the "mother hen" to her teammates. Liz puts the resort and its employees' best interests at the forefront of her daily priorities. Having a resource like Liz and early education programs helped employees better understand and accept their new benefits plan before it was fully implemented.

CASE STUDY:

Great Lakes Auto Network

The Best Benefits Attract the Best Talent

Joey Huang is a career shifter. Despite graduating from dental school and coming from a family of physicians, he opened up a car dealership, Great Lakes Auto Network (GLAN).

Huang's first location is down the street from his father's practice. And he couldn't completely escape the health care industry. As a small business owner, he was tasked with the problem of how to improve and lower the cost of his employee health insurance plan.

The majority of Huang's employees make under $50,000 a year. Asking households to hand over $1,300 or $1,400 every month for health care that didn't meet their expectations wasn't received as a valuable benefit.

But Huang is a strategic businessman, researching other profitable businesses and learning from their successes. He knew that offering better benefits at a low cost would attract and retain the best talent, plus add an extra bonus of saving his company money.

His love for researching best business practices and his familial connections to physicians and providers in the Ashtabula, Ohio, area led him to transitioning to a self-funded plan. He enlisted the help of Bryce Heinbaugh, IEN Risk Management managing partner, to implement the transition.

Prioritizing Transparency

If you're an employer who currently has an advisor that doesn't fight to disclose every fee and cost, including their own compensation, I recommend finding a new one. IEN advisors help employers remodel their plans using Health Rosetta principles, which focus on value-based care and complete transparency of costs in every avenue of health care.

Ethical advisors, ones like Heinbaugh, believe they have a fiduciary responsibility to their plan sponsor, working in the employer's best interest by laying out every cost.

Great employers, like Huang, have the same transparent relationship with their employees. Before changing plans, Huang hosted meetings and sent out educational material about the new benefits plan to resolve confusion among employees who were skeptical of the change.

After the first year of transitioning GLAN to a self-funded plan, Heinbaugh reduced its health care spending by 38%. It managed its costs so well, that GLAN underspent what it estimated to pay for the year and received a claims reimbursement for $138,000. This allowed GLAN to double the size of its workforce and open new locations, expanding from three to six dealerships.

Like any good businessman, Huang reinvested these savings back into his company and shared the wealth with his employees. Employees' cost for family coverage dropped to $980.

Huang added new employee benefits like hosting "health care holiday months" when employees don't have to pay premiums for the month. He also gives employees two options of medical coverage along with valuable add ons, with choices for dental, vision, short-term and long-term disability, voluntary life insurance, accident, and catastrophic coverage.

Heinbaugh connected Huang with services that help GLAN employees navigate the health care landscape, such as the Concierge Nurse Navigator Program that gives employees access to a nurse who acts as a patient advocate. The nurse helps employees schedule appointments, making sure they choose in-network clinicians and hospitals.

Huang credits his industry-leading benefits plan for why he attracts the top talent in the area. Lower costs, better benefits, and improved talent acquisition, what's not to love?

That is why it's always astounding to me when I meet employers who are reluctant or skeptical of changing their health care plan. But my hope is that once they hear enough stories like Heinbaugh's and Huang's they will change their mind and realize that overpaying for subpar insurance is *not* the only option.

CASE STUDY:

Keystone Technologies

Educating Employees to Reduce Your Healthcare Expenses

Growing companies who increase the size of their workforce are rewarded with the benefits of increased productivity and more business opportunities. But more employees comes with a greater responsibility for employers to provide better employee benefits, without pushing their bottom lines.

It's a challenge that Keystone Technologies, a small but quickly growing company from Eureka, Missouri, was struggling to do, as its health care costs continued to grow with every new employee they hired.

The irony is that Keystone is a health care IT firm that provides cyber and computing solutions to hospitals, health systems, and senior-living communities. And even though they specialize in IT services that increase the efficiency and security of health care companies, they were struggling with how to properly manage their own health care benefits.

Keystone is an upsetting example of how all companies, even those working in the health care space, are victims of the inefficiencies and predatory practices of our dysfunctional health care system.

Under its incumbent plan, it was facing a 55% cost increase from its insurance provider and spending 62% above premiums collected (162% loss ratio). The incumbent plan's lack of transparency made it difficult to see where the money was going or what the costs would be, from year to year.

In my experience, these are the types of plans that disempower employers, make them feel helpless to combat rising health care costs, and perpetuate profit-driven incentives in the health care industry.

But fortunately, Keystone is part of the growing number of employers who put their foot down and reject the status quo of low-quality, high-cost health benefits. It had a vision for a new health care plan: one where costs were lower, employee paychecks were higher, and access to health care services could be free.

Its determination to find a solution and keep the business alive led it to Health Rosetta advisor Adam Berkowitz, the founder and president of St. Louis, Missouri-based Simpara Benefits, who guided the company to achieving its dream for a better future.

Within one year, Berkowitz helped Keystone reduce spending by 10%, and by the second year with the new plan, spending dropped 25%. Yearly costs per employee were reduced from $12,000 (PEPY) to $9,441 (PEPY).

Berkowitz managed costs by switching Keystone over to a self-funded plan that incorporated a budget-friendly, maximum-funded plan, where Keystone pays for its maximum liability of claims costs on a monthly basis. Under this new plan, if covered claims are less than what the employer paid for, then the employer receives a refund for unused claim liability at the end of every year. And since changing plans, Keystone has a return worth $60,000, an average of $2,000 per employee per year.

If it had stayed with their old plan, Keystone was facing a 62% increase in premiums. It didn't know how to avoid the increase or where it was coming from. Luckily, Keystone had Berkowitz, a true problem solver who discovered that the old plan had Keystone overspending for health insurance. The company was squandering valuable resources with diminishing returns; and this plan was asking it to increase wasteful spending every year.

To combat the increase, Berkowitz unbundled Keystone's health plan, purchasing benefits from a variety of vendors. This increased vendor competition, thereby lowering prices, and improving price transparency for Keystone employees.

So instead of the predicted 62% increase, Berkowitz reduced spending by 40%, providing Keystone ample flexibility and leverage to grow their business without the burden of out-of-control health care costs.

Employees now have access to a plan that covers 100% of their health costs, which has allowed employees to take expensive medication at no cost to the employee. Their deductibles were cut in half, and single employees now pay an annual **$2,500** and families pay **$5,000** – a price well below the national average.

Improving Member Education

One of the most exceptional strategies that Berkowitz devised to keep health care costs down was educating employees and providing the resources so that they could make smart health care decisions for themselves. Having a good plan is only part of the battle.

Keystone improved workforce health and lowered its health care expenses by teaching employees how to make healthy lifestyle choices, how to find the best prices for medicine and services, and the importance of getting second opinions for treatments.

Employees now have access to tools that promote better health outcomes, like an online health care platform that guides users to make better health care choices.

And while I firmly believe that digital tools are *not* the *sole answer* to solving our health care problems, they are incredible supplements that complement a good health care plan by improving how plan members use their health benefits.

For Keystone employees, online health care tools helped them become more comfortable with shopping and increased their understanding of health care costs. These tools prompted employees to share their experiences with their peers (i.e. finding savings on prescriptions and getting low-cost or free procedures) and helped to bolster the idea that employees have the power and responsibility to be wise health care consumers and advocate for their own health.

Berkowitz's work with Keystone is an example of an advisor who took his duties to the next step, by helping individuals realize that they have control over their health care plan. Too many people think the other way around, and are left feeling trapped.

It's not enough to help create efficient health care plans for organizations. We need to empower employers and employees and give them the knowledge and tools to understand their benefits so that they have the power to seek out the best care and say "no" to plans and providers that don't meet their standards.

CASE STUDY:

Pacific Steel & Recycling

*How One Company Reduced Their Health Plan Cost
by $3.6 Million*

Recycling plants like Pacific Steel and Recycling from Great Falls, Montana, help eliminate metal waste from our world by turning used materials into a new, functional product. Nearly 700 employees work from 46 branch locations in the Western United States and Alberta, Canada.

Pacific Steel's CEO Jeff Mullhollin and CFO Tim Culliton confronted an all-too-common problem: Health care spending was too high. And unfortunately, the company's expertise in reducing material waste didn't translate to solving the problem of eliminating wasteful spending in health care.

Starting in the early 2000s, Pacific Steel embarked on a journey to fixing its health care plan.

First, like many other employers, Pacific Steel tried to combat rising health care expenses by pushing more of the cost onto its employees. But Mullhollin and Culliton soon realized that raising deductibles and contributions didn't address the underlying issues, it just caused another problem: It pushed employees off the plan in favor of cheaper alternatives, like their spouse's plan or marketplace insurance or becoming part of the working uninsured.

The company was fully-insured until the mid-2000s; it later switched to a self-funded health plan with a carrier-based PPO network.

But after experiencing a nearly 400% increase in facility costs in the first part of 2013, the manufacturer implemented reference-based pricing (RBP) beginning January 1, 2014. However, the strategy didn't begin to work until two years later, when the USI health care consulting team came on board, according to Culliton.

Mullhollin and Culliton were led to Scott Haas, Erik Davis, and Terry Killilea, PharmD., all senior vice presidents at USI Insurance Services. Haas, Davis and Killilea are principal consultants within USI Insurance Services, providing health care consulting solutions to their clients.

This unique health care consulting practice ran the numbers provided by the company's TPA and found that some things didn't add up. Many areas were identified where Pacific Steel's 160% of Medicare reimbursement rate was working to its advantage and others where it was wasteful spending. Pacific Steel was often overpaying for certain types of care, spending more than what most other PPO networks pay.

The Power of Reference-Based Pricing and Direct Contracts

That's when USI established benchmarks and metrics to analyze Pacific Steel's health plan data. The USI health care consulting practice repriced the historical claims data to Medicare allowed, which determined the cost basis under the PPO plan as well as the first version of RBP implemented January 1, 2014. Through this process, the USI consulting team developed a second generation RBP solution. Pacific Steel ended up going through two failed TPAs. But the new finalized RBP model involved a member advocacy component and a new TPA, one known for its adjudication integrity and process management.

The new model reimburses providers at fairer and more equitable rates relative to the previous RBP system. Pricing now varies by type and place of service, provider and facility. It also recognizes that 85% – 90% of all health care encounters are with ancillary providers, and the rest with facility-based organizations for surgeries or procedures.

Realizing that RBP cannot produce stellar results on its own, Haas views this strategy as part of an umbrella of alternative reimbursement, as the marketplace evolves toward direct contracting arrangements "without the intermediary of a network or carrier in the middle of the relationship."

RBP addresses pricing, but it does not address utilization variance that will occur regardless of payment level of claims. while revised pricing cannot eradicate large claims or control utilization, Haas says the plan will cycle at "a lower cost threshold because of the reduction in claims cost, which primarily is reflective of a reduction in facility cost."

Pacific Steel now has more than 5,000 safe-harbor or direct contract agreements with high quality physicians and ancillary providers who have agreed not to balance-bill members. This creates an open-access environment, where care essentially can be sought from any provider that Pacific Steel has five direct contracts with and from hospitals and health systems that are based on revised pricing methodology agreements, and others are pending.

USI has also implemented a number of surgical case rates that lead to savings for the plan and the member by paying hospitals, providers, and clinicians a single pre-negotiated rate, instead of billing individually. These contracts pay the provider at the point of service and waive all out-of-pocket cost to the member. Haas negotiated rates for common procedures like hip, joint, and knee replacements. Under Pacific Steel's contract, a knee replacement at designated providers costs around $20,000 – under most plans this procedure can cost upwards of $50,000.

Part of setting those pre-negotiated rates was also doing the research to find the quality providers that practice valued-based care. Pacific Steel has an HR representative who works to match employees with the best clinicians. It encourages its employees to seek out the providers that offer the best care for the most value, incentivizing them to use these providers by waiving the copay. This reduces the number of repeat visits and prevents unnecessary treatment and prescriptions.

Conversely, the company deters employees from going to lower-value providers by informing them that they will have to share the cost for receiving out-of-network care. Being up front about coverage also helps prevent surprise medical bills.

In addition to the cost reduction of the medical plan, the USI health care consulting practice reduced the PBM spend for prescription drugs by over $200,000 in the first year of the revised program. And since 2014, the cost basis of absent specialty-drug utilization has remained flat.

Haas builds plans using Health Rosetta principles. And every plan that incorporates them has what's called the Health Rosetta Dividend, where improving health benefits and lowering costs results in improvement in other areas.

It has made a significant difference at Pacific Steel. The per employee per month composite medical spend, excluding prescription drugs, plummeted 46.1% between the end of 2013 and 2018, falling to $442.32 from $812.13. "That calculates out to an aggregate cost reduction of about $3.6 million," Haas reports.

For Pacific Steel, which has an Employee Stock Ownership Plan – (ESOP) – meaning employees are shareholders of the company – when the company does well or saves money, employees see that success too.

While it took a long time for Pacific Steel to find the right plan and cut costs stories like this should comfort employers, because they show that it's never too late to make a change.

CASE STUDY:

City of Milwaukee

City Slashes Health Care Costs by Improving Benefits

By John Torinus

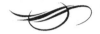

Because the economic pain of out-of-control medical costs are so high and federal government reforms are so slow, school districts, counties, and municipalities are moving on their own to find savings across the four major platforms for containing health care spending: self-insurance, consumer-driven incentives and disincentives, onsite proactive primary care, and value-based purchasing.

The city of Milwaukee, Wisconsin, with 6,500 employees, is one spectacular example. The city has held its health care costs *flat* for the last five years, stopping its previous hyper-inflationary trend of 8%-9% annual increases. Milwaukee spent $139 million on health care in 2011 before switching over to a self-insured plan in 2012. Costs dropped to $102 million in 2012 and have stayed at about that level ever since – even in the face of 6% annual inflation for employer plans nationally over the same period.

If the old trend had continued, health costs for 2016 would have been about $200 million, double what they actually were.

Instead, the cost savings have had many additional positive ramifications: raises for county employees, no layoffs, flat employee premium contributions, better health outcomes for employees and their families, improved productivity, lower absenteeism, and less pressure to raise taxes.

Michael Brady, benefits manager, led this intelligent management approach in close collaboration with the mayor, city council, and unions. As with other enlightened group plans, there are many moving parts. Here's a sampling:

- An onsite wellness center and workplace clinic, headed by nurse practitioners, has sharply reduced hospital admissions. Onsite physical therapy was added last year. These services are free for employees and spouses.
- Relatively low deductibles (now $750 per single employee and $1,500 per family) were installed to create a consumer-friendly environment.
- Coinsurance was set at 10% for members who use United Healthcare's Premium Provider program, which uses only doctors designated as top doctors by UnitedHealthcare. Coinsurance is 30% for providers outside that group. This tiered approach, aimed at improving health outcomes, is a form of value-based purchasing.
- Participants in the city's wellness program can earn $250 in a health account. Good progress has been made on hypertension and smoking (now 12% vs. U.S. average of 14%), but, as with other employers, there's not been as much traction on obesity. There have been some improvements on chronic disease management of diabetes.
- While workplace wellness programs typically have no or negative ROI (see chapter 8's section on this), approaches that use solid clinical evidence to address costly chronic illness and procedures without encouraging overtreatment are sometimes lumped into the same category as typical workplace wellness programs. However, they are highly different in goals, execution, and results.
- A $200 ER copay has cut non-urgent ER visits by 300 per year.
- An intense program to reduce injuries, started in 2008, has resulted in a 70% drop in work hours lost to injury. The program has saved $10 million per year compared to the previous trend line.
- Milwaukee now spends about $15,000 per employee per

year, well below the national average and not too far off the $13,000 at the best private companies.

Government entities are not known for bold innovation, so this track record is an eye-opener, especially in a unionized environment. "The results," said Brady, "are nothing short of amazing considering changes in the city's workforce demographics and the challenging environmental hazards that city employees regularly face."

These changes have taken place at the same time that the nation as a whole has experienced much more disappointing progress from federal reforms (e.g., much higher deductibles for plans sold on ACA exchanges, double-digit premium rises for employers in many states, and a cost to the federal government of about $5,000 per subsidized plan member per year).

Clearly, most of the meaningful reform of the economic chaos from health care in this country is coming from self-insured employers, like the city of Milwaukee.

John Torinus is chairman of Serigraph Inc., a Wisconsin-based graphics parts manufacturer, and author of The Company That Solved Health Care.

CASE STUDY:

Enovation Controls

A Small Oklahoma Manufacturer Removes 97% of Pricing Failure

When you think of innovative organizations that provide a best-of-breed health benefits package and spend far less than peer organizations, you wouldn't necessarily think of small manufacturers in Oklahoma, where as much as 75% of the population doesn't have an established primary care relationship. Yet Enovation Controls, a provider of products and services for engine-driven equipment management and control solutions with about 600 employees, has managed to save approximately $4,000 per covered life each year by working with a transparent open network (TON).

A TON puts together a network of the highest-value providers for different kinds of care and gives self-insured employers a set of fair and fully transparent pricing – typically a bundled price – for medical services/procedures ranging from a specific treatment (e.g., knee replacement or coronary stent) to a specific condition (e.g., diabetes or kidney disease) across multiple providers, and sometimes, multiple settings.

Enovation Controls chose The Zero Card to manage their TON. They achieved a 70% participation rate among eligible plan members, focusing on high-cost services like surgeries and imaging. Justin Bray, Enovation's vice president for organizational effectiveness and human resources, attributes the high rate to two primary factors:

1. **Communications** – During the rollout of the TON, Enovation shared their current health care costs with employ-

ees, along with the consequences for the company and each individual. They then compared those costs with the costs of care under specific scenarios with TON. The message: We've found a better way. Most people were shocked by the vast price disparity and the fact that lower-priced providers often delivered the highest quality, in part because these doctors perform a given procedure more frequently, improving with repetition, which lets them operate efficiently with fewer errors and expensive complications.

2. **Ease of Use** – Employees have access to a single app or phone number that directs them to network providers where they can get care with zero out-of-pocket costs. Instead of dealing with a mountain of bills and paperwork following the procedure, they receive a thank you survey to ensure the experience went well. As Bray explained, this is particularly critical as surgeries and imaging are some of the highest-cost items they have to cover. Because of the focus on higher-cost items, Enovation has achieved well over 90% of projected savings, even with less than 100% participation. The calculation of those potential savings compared the historic "allowable" amount from the company's claims history with a true market amount through the TON network – that is, what a provider would accept if you showed up with a bag of cash for a bundled procedure such as a total knee replacement.

The savings over historical allowable amounts from their traditional PPO network ranged from 21.92% to 81.28%, with an average of 59.23%.

Here's an example of a line item for one procedure for one employee:

"Spinal fusion except cervical without major complications"

Bray shared what this meant to one employee who came up to him at a high school football game to say thank you. This person had recently had expensive surgery and didn't have to pay a dime out of pocket – no bills, no explanations of benefits, no anything. On a $30,000 salary, the maximum allowable out-of-pocket cost of $2,500 under the previous health plan would have been a financial disaster, the employee said.

Enovation Controls Employee Monthly Premium Costs

Historic allowed amount	$129,138
TON network	$38,000
Savings	$91,138

Figure 19: Summary information provided by Enovation Controls.

Like every other health care purchaser, Enovation Controls knows that tackling high-cost procedures is central to slaying the health-care-cost beast. Its TON program even extends to items like complex cardiac and neurosurgical procedures, for which employees have access to the same centers of excellence as large employers, such as Mayo Clinic. Whether the Mayo Clinic or a local surgery center, high-quality providers are happy to provide a deep discount in return for more business, less hassle, and avoiding claims processing and collections processes. Once the procedure is complete, the provider gets paid within five days for the full bundled price.

Plus, the bundled prices frequently carry warranties, meaning postsurgical complications within 60 to 90 days are addressed at no charge – another bonus for employers.

Using data from Mercer, Enovation Controls estimates that they save $2 million on health care every year, compared with peer manufacturing organizations. For a relatively small company, this is a highly meaningful amount of money, which it has been able to reallocate to increased R&D. While companies in their sector typically spend 4% of annual revenues on R&D, Enovation spends 9%, helping it stay ahead of the competition and attract and retain the best engineers.

Enovation Controls Per Capita Spending

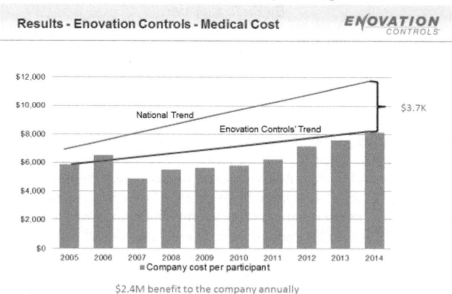

Figure 20: Summary information provided by Enovation Controls.

When a small manufacturer with few dedicated resources can pull this off, it begs the question why every employer or union isn't doing the same. Smart employers like Enovation Controls demonstrate that it's possible, even in a state with some of the highest obesity rates and overall health care costs. Since a new primary care model or TON can be implemented at any point in a benefits cycle, there's no need to wait.

CASE STUDY:

Langdale Industries

A Rural Wood Products Company in a One-Hospital Town Saves Hugely While Ensuring Great Care

By Brian Klepper

L arge American businesses with tens or hundreds of thousands of employees have recruited high-profile benefits profession- als to orchestrate sophisticated campaigns focused on the health of employees and their families – and on the cost-effectiveness of their programs. Even so, few large firms provide comprehensive, quality benefits at a cost that remains consistently below national averages.

For midsized businesses – firms with 100 to 5,000 employees – the task is significantly more difficult without the right peo- ple and focus. Health benefits managers in these companies have far fewer resources, typically work alone without the benefit of a large staff, and are often overwhelmed by the complexity of their tasks. As a result, they often default to whatever their broker and health plan suggest.

But some excel. For them, managing the many different issues – chronic disease, patient engagement, physician self- referrals, specialist and inpatient overutilization, pharmacy management – is a discipline. Barbara Barrett is one of them.

Barrett is director of benefits at TLC Benefit Solutions, Inc., the benefits management arm of Valdosta, Georgia-based Lang- dale Industries, Inc., a small conglomerate of 24 firms and 1,000 employees. Langdale is engaged primarily in producing wood products for the building construction industry, but is also in car dealerships, energy, and other industries.

Valdosta is rural, which puts health benefits programs at a disadvantage. Often, as in this case, there is only one hospital nearby, which means little if any cost competition. Compared with those living in urban areas, rural Georgians are more likely to be less healthy and suffer from heart disease, obesity, diabetes, and cancer. So, the situation is far from ideal.

And yet, from 2000, when Barrett assumed responsibility for the management of Langdale's employee health benefits – to 2009, per employee costs rose from $5,400/year to $6,072/year. That's an average increase of 1.31% per year, compared to an average annual increase of 8.83% for comparably-sized firms nationally. To put this in context, average firms spent $29 million more than Langdale from 2000 to 2009 to provide the same kind of coverage. Langdale's savings were $29,000 per employee – all without reducing the quality of benefits or transferring the cost burden to employees.

Langdale Industries - Actual Premium* vs. US Trend and Cumulative Difference					
Year	US Trend**	Langdale (US Trend)	Langdale Actual***	Diff	Diff x 1,000 EEs
2000		$5,400	$5,400		
2001	11.2%	$6,005	$5,471	$534	$534,060
2002	14.0%	$6,845	$5,542	$1,303	$1,303,065
2003	12.6%	$7,708	$5,615	$2,093	$2,092,989
2004	10.1%	$8,487	$5,689	$2,798	$2,797,941
2005	9.7%	$9,310	$5,763	$3,547	$3,546,612
2006	5.0%	$9,775	$5,839	$3,937	$3,936,601
2007	5.7%	$10,332	$5,915	$4,417	$4,417,301
2008	6.0%	$10,952	$5,993	$4,960	$4,959,756
2009	5.6%	$11,566	$6,071	$5,495	$5,494,583
* For Medical, Dental & Pharmacy			Cumulative Difference		$ 29,082,906
** Source - Kaiser/HRET 2009 Employer Health Benefits Annual Survey					
***Trended at an average of 1.31% between 2000 and 2009					*Brian Klepper*

Figure 21:

So how did Barrett approach the problem? Here are a few of her strategies:

- Langdale set up TLC Benefit Solutions, a HIPAA-compliant firm that administers and processes the company's medical, dental, and drug claims. This allows Barrett to more directly track, manage, and control claim overpayments, waste, and abuse.

- It also gives her immediate access to quality and cost data on doctors, hospitals, and other vendors. Supplementing this data with external information, like Medicare cost reports for hospitals in the region, has allowed her to identify physicians and hospital services that provide low or high value. She has created incentives that steer individuals to high-value physicians and services and away from low-value ones. When necessary complex services are not available locally or have low quality or value, she shops the larger region, often sending patients to higher value centers as far away as Atlanta, three and a half hours by car.

- Barrett analyzes claims data to identify which individuals have chronic disease and which are likely to have a major acute event over the next year. Individuals with chronic diseases are directed into the company's evidence-based, opt-out disease management and prevention program. Individuals with acute care needs are connected with a physician for immediate intervention.

- Langdale provides employees and their families with confidential health advocate services that explain and encourage the use of the company's benefits programs, again using targeted incentives to reward those who enter the programs and meet evidence-based targets.

These are just a few of Barrett's initiatives in group health, but her responsibilities also extend to life insurance, flex plan, supplemental benefits, retirement plan, workers' compensation, liability, and risk insurance. The results for Langdale in these areas include lower than average absenteeism, disability costs, and turnover costs.

The point isn't that you should just do what Barrett and Langdale have done. The point is that they've been proactive, endlessly innovative, and aggressive about managing the process. This attitude and rigor has paid off through tremendous savings, yes, but it has also produced a corporate culture that demonstrates the value of Langdale's employees and community. Employees and their families are healthier as a result and are more productive at work. This has borne unexpected fruit: The industries Langdale is in were hit particularly hard by the recession, and the benefits savings from Barrett's efforts helped save jobs.

Barbara Barrett and many others like her on the front line are virtually unknown in health care. Most often, their achievements go unnoticed beyond the executive offices. But they manage the health care and costs of populations in a way that all groups can be managed.

Editor's note: We checked in with Barbara recently and found that, even in the face of new challenges, such as extreme jumps in drug prices, Langdale continues to succeed where others have failed to carefully manage health costs.

Brian Klepper, PhD, is a health care analyst and principal of Worksite Health Advisors, based in Orange Park, Florida.

CASE STUDY:

Pittsburgh (Allegheny County) Schools

Investing in Kids while Ensuring Teachers Receive Better Care

Bucking old habits that are devastating education funding elsewhere, forward-looking teacher union and school board leaders in Allegheny County, Pennsylvania, are proving that it's not really so difficult to slay the health-care-cost beast and save their kids' future – even in an expensive and contentious health care market. Understandably, unions want their members to be compensated fairly and to keep schools from being decimated. Recognizing that they share the same goals, the school board decided to take a new approach.

Assuming the current trend continues, kindergartners entering Pittsburgh-area schools will collectively have $2 billion more available to invest in education and services over the course of their school years than their counterparts across the state in Philadelphia. In Philadelphia, schools pay $8,815 per member for teacher health benefits. The Allegheny County Schools Health Insurance Consortium (ACSHIC), with 48,000 covered lives, pays $4,661 per member – $199 million less per year. Class sizes in Pittsburgh are 30% smaller, teachers are paid better with better benefits, and there are four times as many librarians.

Rewarding Wise Decisions

Jan Klein, ACSHIC's business manager, describes a model that is very consistent with the Health Rosetta blueprint. In a nutshell, they make smart decisions free or nearly free (e.g., primary care is free, and going to high-quality care providers involves very low or no copays or deductibles) and poor decisions expensive (e.g., paying more to see higher-cost, lower-quality care providers). It's a much more subtle, yet more effective, strategy than blunt-instrument, high-deductible plans that often lead to deferred care, bankruptcies, reduced teacher compensation, fewer arts programs ... the list goes on.

The consortium is managed by 24 trustees, equal parts labor and management. When consultants attend consortium meetings, they often can't tell who is who. Many times, union leaders are more aggressive in pushing forward new initiatives. While other employers have blithely accepted 5% to 20% annual health care cost increases, the consortium spent $233 million in annual claims in 2016 – down from $241 million in 2014. The consortium is able to manage their costs without any stop-loss insurance because they have control over what they call their benefit grid, a program that was defined and embraced by both union leaders and teachers.

They've accomplished this, even though care-provider-organization consolidation in Western Pennsylvania has reduced competition and raised health care costs with little to no improvement in quality of care – and despite an ongoing war between the largest hospital, the University of Pittsburgh Medical Center (UPMC), and the largest local insurance carrier, Highmark.

Understanding that the best way to spend less is to improve health care quality, ACSHIC found that the path began with the following steps:

- Educating consortium trustees on quality rankings of hospitals, including sending them to a Pittsburgh Business Group on health forum
- Retrieving hospital quality data through third-party data and tools (e.g., Imagine Health, CareChex, and Innovu)
- Validating vendor information by confirming it was not influenced by bias
- Selecting the most effective resources by identifying credible partners/vendors

Once educated, the trustees provided the following direction to the team developing the new school district health plan:

- Use quality measures from respected third-party sources.
- Create tiered products so people are free to go wherever they want for care – but they pay more if they choose sites that have lower quality and value.
- Focus on ease of access to regional clinics and hospitals.
- Focus on the relationship between cost and quality (the former turned out not to be indicative of the latter).
- Educate members, especially about why the local academic medical center was placed in a high-cost tier (it wasn't the highest-quality facility for many kinds of care).
- Address member concerns (e.g., Will this really save money?) through continuous communication.

Results

Health care purchasing before (October 2013 - September 2014)

# 1 Hospital in the region (highest quality rating)	#23 Hospital in the region (low quality rating)
33,352 Services*	31,047 Services
293 Admits	362 Admits
$4,941,146 in total costs	$15,089,972 in total costs

Services include imaging, lab tests, outpatient procedures, etc.

Intervention to improve value: tiered benefit offerings

- The enhanced tier has NO deductible and pays 100% of hospital charges.
- The standard tier has a deductible and pays 80% of hospital charges.
- Out-of-network care has a larger deductible and pays 50% of hospital charges.
- Lower cost and higher quality is determined by third-party, independent benchmarks.

Health care purchasing after (October 2015 - September 2016)

#1 Hospital in the region (highest quality rating)	#23 Hospital in the region (low quality rating)
40,046 Services (up 20%)	6,620 Services (down 79%)
328 Admits (up 12%)	113 Admits (down 69%)
$7,170,357 in total costs (up 45%)	$5,548,832 in total costs (down 63%)

Services include imaging, lab tests, outpatient procedures, etc.

In sum, the consortium reduced hospital spending by $7.36 million, a 36.8% reduction.

Going Forward

The consortium expects to continue enhancing benefits with only a very modest premium increase of 1.9% for members. Here are a few plan attributes going forward:

- The enhanced tier has no deductibles.
- Primary care visits have no copay.
- Specialist visits have a $10 copay.
- There's an employee assistance program provider.
- There's a second opinion service.

Their determination to serve kids led education leaders in Pittsburgh to move past tired assumptions about labor and management being forever at odds over health benefits. With any luck, their steely resolve in the face of local challenges will inspire teachers' unions and school boards throughout the country to say "no" to health care stealing our kids' future. Imagine how much better schools would be if every school district replicated Pittsburgh's approach. If you are a parent or community member, share www.healthrosetta.org/schools with leaders in your local schools for this and other examples of success. You can find calculators on how avoiding wasted health care bureaucracy can allow for health and well-being for our future and kids.

CASE STUDY:

Rosen Hotels & Resorts

Smart Benefits Lead to Huge Gains in Education Outcomes and Crime Reduction

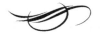

In my experience, speaking with many employers who have slayed the health-care-cost beast, there has been one recurring theme: A leader took the bull by the horns – and did so knowing that success involves weaving employees into the reinvention process rather than trying to pull the wool over their eyes.

Harris Rosen is the founder, COO, and president of Rosen Hotels & Resorts, a small regional chain in Orlando, Florida. Though he's not a health care expert, he intuitively knew what PwC data famously showed: half of health care spending doesn't add value. In a business of ups and downs in which staff costs are a major factor, Rosen surrounded himself with a special executive team to tackle this challenge.

To date, they've adopted more Health Rosetta components than any other company I know, saving approximately $315 million on health care costs since 1971 and spending 50% less per capita than the average employer. If all employers followed suit, we could conservatively remove $500 billion of waste from health care and shift it to more productive sectors of the economy.

Their plan has also grown from 500 to 5,700 lives as the company has grown. They have a very culturally, racially, socio-economically, and demographically diverse employee base, including many immigrants who often haven't had regular access to care before. Yet single coverage for the average employee is only $18.75 per week for benefits that include medical, dental, and pharmacy and, as you'll see below, are better than most of us have ever had.

Rosen also uses focus groups and surveys to match up programs with employee needs, and they continuously refine their programs. Here are a few elements of what makes their program successful:

- They have a comprehensive, onsite 12,000 square-foot medical center that provides access to many routine health care services, far more than typical primary care. They furnished it with used but modern and functional medical equipment for 10 to 15 cents on the dollar. Employees are able to visit the center "on the clock," thus removing a major barrier to receiving care.
- They take great care of individuals, hiring health coaches and nurses to serve as coaches and navigators throughout a medical journey. They use robust, evidence-based approaches to case management, inpatient care management, care transitions, and medication compliance management.
- They have eschewed the blunt instrument approaches most employers use to cut costs (high copays, deductibles) in favor of $5 office visit copays, zero copays for 90% of pharmaceuticals, and no coinsurance. Where necessary, they offer free transportation to appointments to further remove barriers to care.
- Company events serve food approved by nutritionists and the director of health services. They also offer cooking courses.
- They offer the most effective kind of wellness programs for free, including onsite stretching and exercise (e.g., Zumba, kickboxing, walking programs, spinning, boot camp), flu shots and vaccinations, family planning, educational materials, nutritional services, health fairs, and physicals on a schedule informed by the U.S. Preventive Services Task Force, which is far more conservative than the one workplace wellness vendors push.

- They provide free health screenings for colon cancer, diabetes, breast cancer (onsite mammograms), high cholesterol, hypertension, and sexually transmitted diseases, along with visits from registered dietitians. Furthermore, this program follows evidence-based guidelines from organizations like the U.S. Preventive Services Task Force to minimize misdiagnosis and overtreatment.
- Despite physically demanding jobs, onsite physical therapy has led to opioid prescription rates that are one-sixth of the national average.
- They have a mandatory stretching program for housekeepers and other employees with a higher risk of injury, reducing injuries by 25%.
- Fifty-six percent of their employees' pregnancies are high risk, as a result of high rates of advanced maternal age, diabetes, hypertension, and HIV. The company is very proactive about helping employees manage pregnancies (a premature birth can cost $500,000).
- The company cafeteria provides discounts for healthier foods to reduce consumption of unhealthy foods (e.g., discounts on salads). The dietitian and director of health services analyze employee cafeteria offerings for portion size and nutritional benefit. They also use signage to educate employees about nutrition, use smaller plates to control portion sizes, and limit fried foods.
- They focus on better management of chronic conditions and have even seen a drop in the development of new chronic conditions. This is especially important for workers coming from developing countries who often have complex diseases.

Rosen is partnering with other businesses in their community to expand this approach, demonstrating that it's worth ruffling a few feathers to gain the dual benefits of lower costs and a healthier, more satisfied workforce. The ripple effects extend well beyond the company, boosting employee well-being and their broader community's economy. For example, in an industry that sees employee turnover approaching 60%, Rosen has turnover in the low teens.

Rosen pays for full-time employees' college tuition after five years of employment. They also pay state college tuition for employees' children after just three years of employment.

They've also used money that would have been overspent on health care to fuel a range of creative philanthropy. Rosen started by paying for preschool in the underserved, once crime-ridden Tangelo Park neighborhood in Orlando. He's also continued to fund various programs to help those kids develop, such as paying for their college education in full (tuition, room/board, and books). The results have been breathtaking:

- Crime has been reduced by 63%.
- High school graduation rates went from 45% to nearly 100%.
- College graduation rates are 77% above the national average.

The cost over 24 years of the Tangelo Park program has been $11 million – roughly the amount Rosen saves in one year on health care. Recently Rosen has agreed to adopt another underserved community called Parramore, which is five times the size of Tangelo Park.

For Harris Rosen, the approach is simple: Get involved; care for your people.

CASE STUDY:

Textum

A small North Carolina textile company learns how to set its own prices

Sometimes the best innovations come from the smallest groups. Textum, an industrial fabric manufacturer located outside of Charlotte, North Carolina, is one of those small businesses continuously creating and testing new ideas; with 31 employees, Textum has produced unique solutions for a wide variety of industries, from thermal protection systems for space vehicles, carbon fiber material for bulletproof vests, to fabrics used in carbon-carbon processing.

Textum is used to innovating and excelling at every new challenge it encounters. But, in June 2017, annually rising healthcare bills were one issue that really frustrated and stumped Aaron Feinberg, Textum President and CEO. As a small company, Textum's workforce was like family, and Feinberg, knew that rising healthcare costs were not sustainable for his employees or the business at large.

Feinberg quickly realized that his company needed a new health benefits plan, and also that he couldn't do it alone. So, he enlisted the help of David Contorno, a Health Rosetta advisor who is well known for helping businesses, large and small, across the US, save hundreds of millions in healthcare dollars, to create a health plan that functioned as a living document, one that changed as its members' needs and priorities evolved each year.

First, Contorno put the company in a level-funded plan under a BUCAH carrier to ease into the change process in 2018. Level-funded plans are often referred to as "partially self-funded" plans, as they operate in a similar way to a fully self-funded, employer-optimized plan, but have a lower level of stop-loss coverage, which is what protects employers from large claims. (Level-funded plans work well for small companies that want the cost transparency and the minimal savings that come with self-funded plans, but cannot take on the high claims risk that large companies are able to withstand.)

Textum's level-funded plan had an independent TPA, no PPO network, and all the Health Rosetta principles, which in turn helped Feinburg lower his 2018 healthcare costs by $75,762 for the year, or 32%. But, Contorno and Feinburg decided that there were more changes to be made and more savings to be realized the following year.

NEGOTIATING YOUR OWN RATES WITH DIRECT CONTRACTS

In 2019, Contorno introduced several new changes to the healthcare plan. After looking through Textum's claims data from previous years, Contorno found that Textum had a history struggling with balance-billing issues from one particular sizable provider, which left many employees to deal with surprise medical bills that not only was a burden to them, but resulted in less savings than it could otherwise achieve.

To prevent future surprise bills, Contorno created direct contracts with healthcare providers and hospitals in Charlotte that offered the best treatment. He worked with them to negotiate fair rates and payment methodologies for medical services and treatments using reference-based pricing (paying more than Medicare but less than the average PPO network). Then, Contorno bundled surgical and radiological services, implemented international prescription sourcing for low-cost medication, and had the plan waive all out of pocket expenses for members when they used these services.

Pre-negotiated rates helped Textum employees in a number of ways. It directed them to the best providers, increased cost transparency, and prevented them from incurring unknown costs, and improved patient-provider relationships. But Contorno didn't stop there. Taking transparency to another level, Contorno strove to eliminate personal bias by choosing to be paid on a fee and performance basis instead of a commission-basis.

In sum, these strategies resulted in reducing Textum's healthcare spending beyond what Feinburg expected. Textum employees have not seen an increase in deductibles since embarking on this journey to better healthcare in 2017. The 2018 plan had an expected max cost of $176,000. But thanks to the new cost-saving strategies implemented that year, Textum ended up closing the 2018 plan year paying only $155,000 and its health claims spending was 60% below the amount of premiums collected that year (40% loss ratio). If it had stayed on the previous carrier-based plan, Textum would have suffered a sizable $231,000 in healthcare spending in 2018.

In 2019 Textum's max costs were expected to be $189,000. But, once again, Textum came in under budget, spending just $149,133.

As these numbers so clearly demonstrate, Contorno helped Textum regain control over its healthcare plan. He helped Feinburg realize that employers have the power to negotiate and seek out the quality of care that they know their employees deserve. Unfortunately, not all employers know this, which is why finding the right advisors, like Contorno, who fights for the best interests of members are crucial to transforming the status quo and fixing healthcare.

CASE STUDY:

ETEX Telephone Co-Operative

*A Texas fiber and telecommunications provider joins
the local healthcare movement*

Charlie Cano, CEO and general manager of ETEX – one of the largest telecom co-ops in Gilmer, Texas that provides internet, phone, and TV for over 13,000 customers and numerous school districts in the northeast Texas region – is an engineer by trade. He is accustomed to understanding how things work, but when it came to health insurance, he was wrought with confusion about hidden fees, high cost pharmaceuticals, and constant rate increases.

Paige Mendez is now an Employee Benefits Consulting, LLC (EBC) team member who previously worked at the third-party administrator that manages ETEX's benefit plan. Paige recommended that Charlie talk to Rachel Means, CEO of EBC, who founded the Tyler, Texas firm in 2016 to break away from predatory insurance practices and start an advisory group that strove to provide plan members with the highest-quality, most affordable care.

In an hour-long meeting over lunch, Means took the time to answer each and every one of Cano's questions, demonstrating transparency he had yet to experience from any other advisor. Means told Cano about hidden commissions, fees, and other wasteful spending in his company's plan. After talking, Cano was convinced that Means could help him achieve his goal of creating a better health plan – one his 150 employees deserved.

LOCALIZING CARE

The first thing that Means did to push down ETEX's health spend was change its pharmacy benefits manager (PBM) to one that was more transparent. Means pointed out the pain points in ETEX's health plan, much of which came from several high-cost member medications. Cano, like many employers, believed that the billed prices of medical services and drugs were final, non-negotiable, and due in full. But, Means helped him realize that there is always room for negotiation, and that employers have the power to create strategies to find lower prices while still providing employees with the care and medication they need.

Specifically, Means helped Cano find alternative drug suppliers that cut out inflated drugs costs and administrative fees. Switching to a fiduciary PBM and sourcing prescriptions from manufacturers and low-cost, local pharmacies slashed ETEX's pharmacy costs by 50% and had the added benefit of supporting Means' and Cano's local community. These changes have reduced per employee per year medical and prescription costs by $5,743 a year, since 2017.

Means continued to seek out local, affordable healthcare options for ETEX's primary care services. She set up contracts with direct primary care (DPC) physicians and imaging centers in the northeast Texas regions of Longview and Tyler. ETEX health plan members now have $0 out-of-pocket costs for X-rays, CT scans, MRIs, minor emergency room/urgent care visits, and primary care appointments. Members even have access to $0 diabetic supplies, like insulin, pumps, and meters, plus no-cost hormone replacement therapy.

When employees and their families visit their DPC physician, they don't have to sit in a waiting room for half an hour or more for their appointments. Because the DPC model is based on a membership fee, physicians have more time to listen to patients without time constraints or the pressure of hospital referral quotas to meet. ETEX health plan members enjoy a better patient experience with better outcomes and no out-of-pocket cost.

These changes have not only resulted in better benefits, but also a total savings of $2.5M in three years. ETEX has seen $863,000 in year-over-year savings since 2017.

Employees now have access to $0 high-quality healthcare and Cano has used a portion of the savings to give employee bonuses. ETEX's turnover rate has decreased and Cano has noticed that employee morale has increased since implementing these additional programs. Better healthcare benefits have made ETEX more competitive and appealing to potential hires, Cano even mentioned they have a waiting list of candidates wanting to work for ETEX.

This case study shows why providing your employees with better, more affordable care using local providers is a win-win for you and your community. Big carriers and profit-focused PBMs harm local pharmacies and physicians, and by extracting them from employers' health plans the way Means did for Cano, businesses can not only save money; they can potentially save their local community.

Case Studies

ABOUT THE AUTHOR

D ave Chase is an industry ecosystem thinker and shifter, and the founder of Health Rosetta, an organization that provides a blueprint for high-performance health benefits (healthrosetta. org). Health Rosetta accelerates the adoption of simple, practical, nonpartisan fixes to our health care system. Its guiding principles are inspired by the Cluetrain Manifesto – a major influence on the development of the internet – and written by Chase and Leonard Kish. "The Health Rosetta Principles: Guiding Principles for a New Health Ecosystem" covers a wide variety of topics from medical science to economics to community-driven health, and features essays from leading thinkers like Bill Gates; Shannon Brownlee; Esther Dyson; Rushika Fernandopulle, MD; Susannah Fox; Zayna Khayat, PhD; Daniel Kraft, MD; Eric Topol, MD; and many others.

Health Rosetta was formally launched in September 2017 with the release of Chase's best-selling book, *The CEO's Guide to Restoring the American Dream*, which focuses on how high-performing organizations have solved health care's toughest challenges. His TEDx Talk "Health Care Stole the American Dream Here's How We Take It Back" echoes similar sentiments.

Since the launch of Health Rosetta, over 1,000 benefits brokers have applied to the Health Rosetta program, with just 15% accepted based on a proven track record and/or mission alignment. These benefits advisors are responsible for stewarding nearly five million American lives, and also work with federal

Rehumanizing Health Plans That Restore Health, Hope, and Well-Being and state officials to achieve the quadruple aim and transform health care in their communities.

Recently, Chase acted as a consultant to FOX's *The Resident*, which is reshaping the medical drama genre to address the implications of perverse incentives in status quo care. Already achieving over 10 million weekly viewers in just its second season, The Resident has carved out a niche in a crowded arena. Season *three* takes on the many issues of hospital consolidation that affect the well-being of clinicians and patients alike.

Some of Chase's earlier achievements include co-editing the seminal book on patient engagement, *Engage! Transforming Healthcare Through Digital Patient Engagement*, which won HIMSS book of the year in 2014. He wrote the seminal paper on direct primary care, and as a leader of the industry association for digital advertising (Interactive Advertising Bureau), played a driving role in turning the digital advertising market around in the aftermath of the dotcom bust.

Chase was also the CEO and co-founder of Avado, acquired by and integrated into WebMD and Medscape. Before Avado, Chase spent several years outside of health care working with startups – LiveRez.com, MarketLeader, and WhatCounts – either as a founder or consultant. He also served in leadership roles for two $1 billion-plus businesses within Microsoft, including their $2 billion health care platform business.

Chase is active in social ventures and is a student of social enterprises/movements ranging from sustainable building and microcredit to rural hospital development and the re-creation of the U.S. food system.

Chase is a husband, father of two student athletes, and a high school track and cross country coach. In his first season with the team, the girl's track team won their first state championship in 30 years, with multiple individual state champions and podium finishes. Despite being unranked in preseason polls after losing two star runners, the girls placed second in the state's cross-country championship. Coming into conference champion ships, the boys team was seeded 20th in the state but went on to place 4th in state.

Chase is also a former PAC-12 800-meter competitor and an oxygen-fueled mountain athlete. His team recently placed 3rd in their division and 24th overall (of 500 teams) in the oldest adventure race in the U.S., where Dave tackled the Nordic ski leg.

About the Author

REFERENCES

1   Wayland, Michael. "Auto Analyst Jonas Says Investors 'Comfortable' with GM Strike despite Potential Multibillion Cost." *CNBC*, October 14, 2019. https://www.cnbc.com/2019/10/14/jonas-investors-ok-with-gm-strike-despite-potential-multibillion-cost.html.

2   Chase, Dave. "The GM-UAW Strike Can Teach Us a Thing or Two about Health Care." *BenefitsPRO*, October 24, 2019. https://www.benefitspro.com/2019/10/24/the-gm-uaw-strike-can-teach-us-a-thing-or-two-about-health-care/.

3   CBS Boston. "Dedham Teachers Go On Strike, First Mass. Teachers Strike In 12 Years." *CBS Boston*, October 25, 2019. https://boston.cbslo-cal.com/2019/10/25/dedham-teachers-strike-schools-closed-educators-association-picket-line/.

4   "Defying Injunction, Massachusetts Teachers Strike." Labor Notes, October 25, 2019. https://www.labornotes.org/blogs/2019/10/defy-ing-injunction-massachusetts-teachers-strike.

5   Fordham, Evie. "25,000 University of California Workers to Strike Wednesday." *Fox Business*, November 13, 2019. https://www.foxbusiness.com/money/strike-november-2019-university-california.

6   Bartlett, Jessica. "First Look: MGH Plans 1 Million-Square-Foot Expansion." *Boston Business Journal*, May 13, 2019. https://www.bizjournals.com/boston/news/2019/05/13/first-look-mgh-plans-1-million-square-foot.html.

7   Kowalick, Claire. "Report Finds Texas Has the 10th Highest Obesity Rate in the U.S." *Wichita Falls Times Record News*, September 16, 2019. https://www.timesrecordnews.com/story/news/local/2019/09/12/texas-ranks-10th-obesity-in-america-1-in-3-people-obese/2300871001/.

8   Influence & Lobbying / Lobbying / Top Industries." Open Secrets.org, accessed February 28, 2018, https://www.opensecrets.org/lobby/top. php?indexType=i.

9   "IOM Report: Estimated $750B Wasted Annually in Health Care System." *Kaiser Health News*, accessed July 4, 2016, http://khn.org/morning-breakout/iom-report/; "The Price of Excess, Identifying Waste in Healthcare Spending." PricewaterhouseCoopers Health Research Institute.

10 Kocher, Bob. "How I Was Wrong About ObamaCare." accessed December 11, 2019, https://www.wsj.com/articles/i-was-wrong-about-obamacare-1469997311.

11 Brewers Association. "National Beer Sales & Production Data." accessed December 12, 2019, https://www.brewersassociation.org/sta-tistics-and-data/national-beer-stats/.

12 Morris, Zoë Slote, Steven Wooding, and Jonathan Grant. "The Answer Is 17 Years, What Is the Question: Understanding Time Lags in Translational Research." *Journal of the Royal Society of Medicine*. Royal Society of Medicine Press, December 2011. https://www.ncbi.nlm.nih.gov/pmc/articles/PMC3241518/.

13 Institute for Healthcare Improvement. "Charting the Way to Greater Success: Pursuing Perfect in Sweden." accessed December 12, 2018, http://www.ihi.org/resources/Pages/ImprovementStories/ChartingtheWaytoGreaterSuccessPursuingPerfectioninSweden.aspx.

14 Makary, Marty. "We Spend about Half of Our Federal Tax Dollars on Health Care. That's Ridiculous." *USA Today*. Gannett Satellite Information Network, September 16, 2019. https://www.usatoday.com/story/opinion/2019/09/16/spend-about-half-federal-tax-dollars-health-care-ridiculous-column/2301040001/.

15 Gates, Bill. "How State Budgets Are Breaking US Schools." YouTube. TED, March 4, 2011. https://www.youtube.com/watch?v=jiUK-pX-09zo4.

16 Pohle, Allison. "Boston Public School Students Are Walking out-Again-to Protest the Budget." *Boston Globe*, May 17, 2016. https://www.boston.com/news/education/2016/05/17/boston-public-school-walkout-protest-budget.

17 Rocheleau, Matt. "High Lead Levels Found in Water at Hundreds of Schools." *Boston Globe*, May 2, 2017. https://www.bostonglobe.com/metro/2017/05/01/high-lead-levels-found-hundreds-massachusetts-schools/bflx2ZXaLYLSl10r0Hvj7L/story.html.

18   Massachusetts Nurses Association. "Massachusetts Hospitals Stock- pile $1.6 Billion in Cayman Islands and Other Offshore Accounts; Nurses Call for Financial Transparency." *PR Newswire*. Massachusetts Nurses Association, May 30, 2019. https://www.prnewswire.com/ news-releases/massachusetts-hospitals-stockpile-1-6-billion-in-cay- man-is-lands-and-other-offshore-accounts-nurses-call-for-financial-transparency-300859177.html.

19   Health Policy Commission, "List of Figures in 2013 Cost Trends Report by the Health Policy Commission." Health Policy Com- mis- sion, accessed July 4, 2016, https://www.mass.gov/files/docu-ments/2016/07/pb/2013-ctr-chartbook.pdf

20   Kilpatrick, Tim. "Blame the Healthcare System for Bad Health? Here's 14 Things It Should Change." *MedCity News*, March 29, 2017. http://medcitynews.com/2014/10/14-patient-barriers-may-delay-prevent-re-covery/.

21   Devitt, Michael. "CDC Data Show U.S. Life Expectancy Continues to Decline." *AAFP Home*, December 10, 2018. https://www.aafp.org/news/health-of-the-public/20181210lifeexpectdrop.html.

22   Allen, Marshall. "What Happens When a Health Plan Has No Limits? An Acupuncturist Earns $677 a Session." *ProPublica*, December 19, 2019. https://www.propublica.org/article/what-happens-when-a-health-plan-for-teachers-has-no-limits-an-acupuncturist-earns-677-a-session.

23   Chase, Dave. "What the U.S. Could Buy With Wasted Healthcare Dol-lars." *Forbes*, February 2, 2015. http://www.forbes.com/sites/ da-vechase/2012/10/27/what-the-u-s-could-buy-with-wasted-health care-dollars/.

24   The Sun Newspapers. "Letter to the Editor: Healthcare Costs Drain School Budget." *The Moorestown Sun*, April 12, 2014. http://www.moorestownsun.com/2014/04/11/letter-to-the-editor-health care-costs-drain-school-budget/.

25   Chase, Dave. "Healthcare 'Tax' Has Crushed Nest Eggs By $1,000,000 Per Household." *Forbes*, May 28, 2015. https://www.forbes.com/sites/davechase/2015/05/27/health-care-tax-has-crushed-nest-eggs-by-1000000-per-household.

26   "The Health Rosetta." Health Rosetta. Accessed December 19, 2019. https://healthrosetta.org/health-rosetta/#basics.

27 "At the Epicenter of the COVID-19 Pandemic and Humanitarian Crises in Italy: Changing Perspectives on Preparation and Mitigation." New England Journal of Medicine accessed April 9, 2020 https://catalyst.nejm.org/doi/full/10.1056/CAT.20.0080.

28 Gould, Elise. "2014 Continues a 35-Year Trend of Broad-Based Wage Stagnation." EPI analysis of Current Population Survey Outgoing Rotation Group microdata, Economic Policy Institute, accessed April 27, 2018, https://www.epi.org/publication/stagnant-wages-in-2014/.

29 Graphic courtesy of Dr. Paul Grundy, IBM's Chief Medical Officer and Director of Health Care Transformation IBM Health Care Life Science Industry.

30 Cothran, Josh. "US Health Care Spending: Who Pays?"

31 "How Many Doctors Does It Take to Start a Healthcare Revolution? Full Transcript." Freakonomics, accessed July 4, 2017, http://freakonomics.com/2015/04/09/how-many-doctors-does-it-take-to-start-a-health care-revolution-full-transcript/.

32 Keckley, Paul, PhD. "Keynote: Health Reform 2.0: What's Ahead?" filmed March 2015, 4:02, https://www.youtube.com/watch?v=m4cZ4kZw8-E&fea-ture=youtu.be&t=4m2s.

33 "When a Hospital Closes: What Really Happens to the Patients Left Behind?" *Advisory Board*, accessed November 5, 2017, http://www.advisory.com/daily-briefing/2015/05/06/when-a-hospital-closes-what-really- happens-to-the-patients-left-behind.

34 "Study: 7 of 10 Most Profitable US Hospitals Are Nonprofits." AP News, accessed November 5, 2017, https://apnews.com/8867beb-032c049378e4a83d-150cb8bc3.

35 Herman, Bob. "Hospitals Are Making a Fortune on Wall Street." *Axios*, December 7, 2017. https://www.axios.com/hospitals-are-making-a-for- tune-on-wall-street-1513388345-1b7e1923-e778-4627-8fcc-bfab39e2d5c4. html.

36 Galewitz, Phil and Anna Gorman, "More Ailing Hospitals Are Being Resuscitated as Upscale Living Spaces." *Washington Post*, accessed Decem- ber 7, 2017, https://www.washingtonpost.com/realestate/more-ail-ing-hospitals-are-being-resuscitated-as-upscale-living-spac-es/2017/11/21/ e1af7ec2-b34f-11e7-9e58-e6288544af98_story.html.

37 Kaysen, Ronda. "Repurposing Closed Hospitals as For-Profit Med- ical Malls." *New York Times*, accessed November 5, 2017, https:// www.ny-times.com/2014/03/05/realestate/commercial/repurpos- ing-closed-hospitals-as-for-profit-medical-malls.html.

38   Woodard, Colin. "The Coolest Shipyard in America." Politico Magazine, accessed February 17, 2018, https://www.politico.com/magazine/story/2016/07/philadelphia-what-works-navy-yard-214072.

39   Chase, Dave. "VP HR & Benefits Should Get Big Bonuses for Saving 50-90% on Big Ticket Healthcare." LinkedIn, accessed September 28, 2014, https://www.linkedin.com/pulse/20140928130122-255656-vp-hr-benefits-should-get-big-bonuses-saving-50-90-on-big-ticket-health care/.

40   Fry, Richard. "Millennials Surpass Gen Xers as the Largest Generation in U.S. Labor Force." Pew Research Center, accessed January 18, 2018, http://www.pewresearch.org/facttank/2015/05/11/millennials-surpass-gen-xers-as-the-largest-generation-in-us-labor-force/.

41   Goldhill, David. *Catastrophic Care: Why Everything We Think We Know about Heath Care Is Wrong.* New York: Knopf Doubleday Publishing Group, 2013.

42   Hidalgo, Jason. "Here's How Millennials Could Change Health Care." *USA Today,* accessed February 7, 2018, http://www.usatoday.com/story/news/politics/elections/2016/02/07/heres-how-millenni-als-could-change-health-care/79818756/.

43   "The Future Health Ecosystem Today." Cascadia Capital, accessed January 15, 2016, http://www.cascadiacapital.com/story/cascadias-digital-healt-care-team-releases-the-future-of-health care-today-report/

44   Dimock, Michael. "Defining Generations: Where Millennials End and Generation Z Begins." Pew Research Center. Pew Research Center, January 17, 2019. https://www.pewresearch.org/fact-tank/2019/01/17/where-millennials-end-and-generation-z-begins/.

45   Crichton, Danny. "Millennials Are Destroying Banks, and It's the Banks' Fault." *TechCrunch,* accessed February 15, 2018, https://techcrunch.com/2015/05/30/millennial-banks/.

46   Hanft, Adam. "The Stunning Evolution of Millennials: They've Become the Ben Franklin Generation." THE BLOG *Huffington Post,* accessed January 11, 2017, http://www.huffingtonpost.com/adam-hanft/the-stunning-evolution-of_b_6108412.html.

47   Crichton, Danny. "Millennials Are Destroying Banks, and It's the Banks' Fault."

48   Farr, Christina. "Are Millennials Ready to Ditch Their Regular Doctor?" KQED *Science,* accessed July 4, 2017), http://ww2.kqed.org/futureofyou/2015/08/12/convenience-or-loyalty-what-do-millennials-value-more-when-it-comes-to-their-health.

49   "Growing Retail Clinic Industry Employs, Empowers Nurse Practitioners." Robert Wood Johnson Foundation, accessed July 4, 2016, http://www.rwjf.org/en/library/articles-and-news/2015/02/growing-retail-clinic-industry-employs--empowers-nurse-practitio.html; Pollack, Craig E., et al. "The Growth of Retail Clinics and the Medical Home: Two Trends in Concert or in Conflict?" *Health Affairs* (29): 5, accessed July 4 2016, doi: 10.1377/hlthaff.2010.0089; Jaspen, Bruce. "Retail Clinics Hit 10 Million Annual Visits but Just 2% of Primary Care Market." *Forbes*, accessed July 4, 2016, https://www.forbes.com/sites/brucejaspen/2015/04/23/retail-clinics-hit-10-million-annual-visits-but-just-2-of-primary-care-market.

50   Hidalgo, Jason. "Here's How Millennials Could Change Health Care".

51   "People Love Their Health Benefits. But Do They Understand Them?" *Collective Health* (2016), https://collectivehealth.com/insights/consumer-health-benefits-survey-2015/.

52   Hidalgo, Jason. "Here's How Millennials Could Change Health Care."

53   Dews, Fred. "Brookings Data Now: 75 Percent of 2025 Workforce Will Be Millennials." accessed July 4, 2016, https://www.brookings.edu/blog/brookings-now/2014/07/17/brookings-data-now-75-percent- of-2025-workforce-will-be-millennials/; Mitchell, Alastair. "The Rise of the Millennial Workforce," *Wired*, accessed May 25, 2017, https://www. wired. com/insights/2013/08/the-rise-of-the-millennial-workforce/.

54   "Freelancers Now Make Up 35% Of U.S. Workforce," *Forbes*, accessed June 25, 2018, https://www.forbes.com/sites/elainepofeldt/2016/10/06/new-survey-freelance-economy-shows-rapid-growth.

55   "A Conversation with Surgeon, Author, and Researcher Atul Gawande." Interview by Judy Woodruff. Filmed June 2018 The Aspen Insti- tute - Aspen Ideas Festival, Aspen CO, https://www.youtube.com/watch?v=_kaB8UL_TNk&feature=youtu.be.

56   "Obamacare Plans Get More Restrictive and Deductibles Get Pricier in 2018." CNBC, accessed June 25, 2018, https://www.cnbc.com/2017/11/30/obamacare-plans-get-narrower-and-deductibles-get-pricier-in-2018.html.

57   Chase, Dave. "Healthcare Stole the American Dream - Here's How We Take It Back." YouTube. TEDx Talks, January 4, 2017. https://www.youtube.com/watch?v=wKmbKEOUaQU.

58 Cutter, Chip. "The Opioid Crisis is Creating a Fresh Hell for America's Employers." LinkedIn, accessed December 12, 2019, https://www.linkedin.com/pulse/opioid-crisis-creating-fresh-hell-americas-employers-chip-cutter/.

59 By William Wan and Heather Long 'Cries for help': Drug overdoses are soaring during the coronavirus pandemic https://www.washingtonpost.com/health/2020/07/01/coronavirus-drug-overdose/

60 America's Drug Overdose Epidemic: Data to Action https://www.cdc.gov/injury/features/prescription-drug-overdose/index.html

61 Fain, Kevin M., JD, MPH and G. Caleb Alexander, MD, MS. "Mind the Gap: Understanding the Effects of Pharmaceutical Direct-to-Consumer Advertising." *Medical Care* 52(2014): 4, accessed July 4, 2017, doi: 10.1097/ MLR.0000000000000126.

62 Katz, Josh. "Drug Deaths in America Are Rising Faster Than Ever." *New York Times*, accessed July 4, 2017, https://www.nytimes.com/interactive/2017/06/05/upshot/opioid-epidemic-drug-overdose-deaths-are-ris- ing-faster-than-ever.html.

63 Cutter, Chip. "The Opioid Crisis Is Creating a Fresh Hell for America's Employers," accessed August 4, 2017, https://www.linkedin.com/pulse/opioid-crisis-creating-fresh-hell-americas-employers-chip-cutter/.

64 DeWine, Mike. "Economic Aspects of Opioid Crisis." Filmed June 2017 at Longworth House Office Building, Washington D.C. Video 26:41. https://www.youtube.com/watch?v=LIQIQ1jC2dg&feature=youtu.be&t=1601.

65 Donnelly, Frank. "Staten Island Ferry Ex-Captain Details Chaos That Enveloped Barberi after Fatal Crash," Silive.com, accessed July 4, 2017, http://www.silive.com/news/2010/07/staten_island_ferry_excaptain.html.

66 Meier, Barry. "Pain Pills Add Cost and Delays to Job Injuries." *New York Times*, accessed July 4, 2017, http://www.nytimes.com/2012/06/03/health/painkillers-add-costs-and-delays-to-workplace-injuries.html.

67 Bachhuber, Marcus A., MD, MSHP et al. "Increasing Benzodiazepine Prescriptions and Overdose Mortality in the United States, 1996–2013," *American Journal of Public Health*, April 2016, accessed January 17, 2018, doi: 10.2105/ AJPH.2016.303061.

68   Grohol, John. "Top 25 Psychiatric Medications for 2016." *PsychCentral*, accessed February 14, 2018, https://psychcentral.com/blog/top-25-psychiatric-medications-for-2016/.

69   Ornstein, Charles and Ryann Grochowski Jones. "One Nation, Under Sedation: Medicare Paid for Nearly 40 Million Tranquilizer Prescriptions in 2013" *ProPublica*, accessed January 4, 2018, https://www.propublica.org/article/medicare-paid-for-nearly-40-million-tranquilizer-prescriptions-in-2013.

70   Adi Jaffe PhD., "Alcohol, Benzos, and Opiates – Withdrawal That Might Kill You." *Psychology Today*, accessed December 19, 2019 https://www.psychologytoday.com/us/blog/all-about-addiction/201001/alcohol-benzos-and-opiates-withdrawal-might-kill-you.

71   Kolodny, Andrew et al. "The Prescription Opioid and Heroin Crisis: A Public Health Approach to an Epidemic of Addiction." *Annual Review of Public Health*, 36(2015): 559, accessed July 4, 2017, doi:10.1146/annurev-publhealth-031914-122957.

72   Frieden, Thomas R., MD, MPH, and Debra Houry, MD, MPH. "Reducing the Risks of Relief – The CDC Opioid-Prescribing Guideline." *New England Journal of Medicine* 374 (2016): 1501-1504, accessed July 4, 2017, doi: 10.1056/ NEJMp1515917.

73   Chou, Roger, MD et al. "The Effectiveness and Risks of Long-Term Opioid Therapy for Chronic Pain: A Systematic Review for a National Institutes of Health Pathways to Prevention Workshop." *Annual Internal Medicine* 162 (2015): 4, accessed July 4, 2017, doi: 10.7326/M14-2559.

74   Lembke, Anna, MD; Keith Humphreys, PhD; and Jordan Newmark, MD. "Weighing the Risks and Benefits of Chronic Opioid Therapy." *American Family Physician*, accessed July 4, 2017 www.aafp.org/afp/2016/0615/p982.html.

75   Fain, Kevin M., JD, MPH and G. Caleb Alexander, MD, MS. "Mind the Gap: Understanding the Effects of Pharmaceutical Direct-to-Consumer Advertising." *Medical Care* 52 (2014): 4, accessed July 4, 2017, doi: 10.1097/MLR.0000000000000126.

76   Freburger, Janet K., PT, PhD, et al. "Rising Prevalence of Chronic Low Back Pain." *Arch Intern Med.* 169(2009): 3, accessed July 4, 2017, doi: 10.1001/archinternmed.2008.543.

77   Monnat, Shannon. "Deaths of Despair and Support for Trump in the 2016 Presidential Election." The Pennsylvania University Department of Agricultural Economics, Sociology, and Education Research Brief, accessed July 4, 2017. http://aese.psu.edu/directory/smm67/Elec- tion16.pdf.

78   Hollingsworth, Alex, Christopher J. Ruhm, and Kosali Simon. "Macro- eco- nomic Conditions and Opioid Abuse." The National Bureau of Eco- nomic Research, accessed July 4, 2017, http://www.nber.org/papers/w23192.

79   "Bureau of Labor Statistics for 2016." Social Security Administration, accessed October 24, 2017, https://www.ssa.gov/cgi-bin/netcomp. cgi?-year=2016.

80   Rabin, Roni Caryn. "15-Minute Visits Take a Toll on the Doctor-Pa- tient Relationship." accessed December 29, 2017, https://khn.org/ news/15-minute-doctor-visits.

81   Viadro, Christopher. "Increase in Opiate Usage Appears Tied to De- crease in Access to Treatment in Worker's Compensation." Butler-Viadro, LLP, accessed July 4, 2017, http://www.butlerviadro.com/ blog/2016/05/increase-in-opiate-usage-appears-tied-to-decrease-in-ac- cess-to-treatment-in-workers-com- pensation.shtml.

82   Chase, Dave. "City Slashes Healthcare Costs by Improving Health Benefits." Forbes, February 8, 2016, accessed July 4, 2017, https://www. forbes.com/sites/davechase/2016/02/08/city-slashes-health care-costs-by-improving- health-benefits.

83   Connor, Vickie. "Patients with Mental Disorders Get Half of All Opioid Prescriptions." accessed July 4, 2017, http://khn.org/news/patients- with-mental-disorders-get-half-of-all-opioid-prescriptions/.

84   Fenton, Joshua J. MD, MPH et al. "The Cost of Satisfaction: A National Study of Patient Satisfaction, Health Care Utilization, Expenditures, and Mortality." Arch Intern Med. 172(2012): 5, accessed July 4, 2017, doi: 10.1001/archinternmed.2011.1662.

85   Fenton, Joshua J., MD, MPH et al. "The Cost of Satisfaction: A National Study of Patient Satisfaction, Health Care Utilization, Expenditures, and Mortality."

86   Robbins, Rebecca. "Do Americans Really Watch 16 Hours of Pharma Ads a Year?," STAT News, accessed September 12, 2017, https://www. statnews.com/2017/09/12/americans-16-hours-pharma-ads/.

87   "New Research Reveals the Trends and Risk Factors Behind America's Growing Heroin Epidemic." CDC, accessed July 4, 2017, https://www. cdc.gov/media/releases/2015/p0707-heroin-epidemic.html.

88   Roy, Avik. "If Republicans Delay the Cadillac Tax, They Will Cost Taxpay- ers Far More in the Long Run." Forbes, accessed March 26, 2018, https:// www.forbes.com/sites/theapothecary/2015/12/11/if-repub- licans-de- lay-the-cadillac-tax-they-will-cost-taxpayers-far-more-in-the- long-run.

89   "Health Care Costs: A Primer." The Henry J. Kaiser Family Foundation, accessed July 4, 2016, http://www.kff.org/report-section/health-care-costs-a-primer-2012-report/.

90   Sussman, Anna Louie. "Burden of Health-Care Costs Moves to the Middle Class." *Wall Street Journal*. Dow Jones & Company, August 25, 2016. https://www.wsj.com/articles/burden-of-health-care-costs-moves-to-the-middle-class-1472166246

91   Pinder, Jeanne. "Cash Prices Stay Level, While Overall Costs Continue to Rise." *Clear Health Costs*, April 1, 2017. https://clearhealthcosts.com/blog/2017/03/cash-prices-stay-level-overall-costs-continue-rise/.

92   "Fraud, Waste and Abuse in Social Services: Identifying and Overcoming This Modern-Day Epidemic." Accenture Consulting.

93   Rayman, Noah. "The World's Top 5 Cybercrime Hotspots." *Time*, accessed July 4, 2016, http://time.com/3087768/the-worlds-5-cybercrime-hotspots/.

94   Rashid, Fahmida. "Why Hackers Want Your Health Care Data Most of All." *InfoWorld*, accessed July 4, 2016, http://www.infoworld.com/article/2983634/security/why-hackers-want-your-health-care-data-breaches- most-of-all.html.

95   *The Nilson Report* (October 2016): 1096, accessed January 17, 2017, https://www.nilsonreport.com/upload/content_promo/The_Nil- son_Report_10-17-2016.pdf; Kiernan, John. "Credit Card & Debit Card Fraud Statistics." *WalletHub*, accessed March 2, 2017, https://wallethub. com/edu/credit-debit-card-fraud-statistics/25725/.

96   Private discussions by the author with other industry executives and experts, not for attribution.

97   "Fiduciary Responsibilities." U.S. Department of Labor. Accessed December 18, 2019. https://www.dol.gov/general/topic/health- plans/fiduciaryresp.

98   Mitchell, Jerry and (Jackson, Miss.) Clarion Ledger. "Opioid Mak- ers Face Hundreds of Lawsuits for Misleading Doctors about Drug's Addictive Nature." *USA Today*, accessed March 26, 2018, https://www.usatoday.com/story/news/nation-now/2018/01/29/judge-stop-legal-fights-and-curb-opioid-epidemic/1072798001/.

99   "The Underestimated Cost of the Opioid Crisis." The Council of Economic Advisers, accessed March 20, 2018, https://www.whitehouse.gov/sites/whitehouse.gov/files/images/The%20Underestimated%20Cost%20of%20 the%20Opioid%20Crisis.pdf.

100 "The $272 Billion Swindle: Why Thieves Love America's Health-Care System." *The Economist,* accessed March 26, 2018, https://www.economist.com/news/united-states/21603078-why-thieves-love-americas-health-care- system-272-billion-swindle.

101 "A Substance Use Cost Calculator for Employers." National Safety Council, accessed March 20, 2018, https://forms.nsc.org/substance-use-employer-calculator/index.aspx.

102 Goplerud, Eric, Sarah Hodge, and Tess Benham. "A Substance Use Cost Calculator for US Employers with an Emphasis on Prescription Pain Medication Misuse." *Journal of Occupational and Environmental Medicine,* 2017 Nov, 59(11): 1063–1071.https://dx.doi.org/10.1097%2F JOM.0000000000001157.

103 "Medication Assisted Treatment & Direct Primary Care." Bluegrass Family Wellness, accessed March 20, 2018, http://www.bluegrassfamilywellness.com/home-recovery/.

104 "Vera Whole Health Achieves Validation Endorsement by Care InnovationsTM Validation Institute." accessed April 27, 2018, https://www.prnewswire.com/news-releases/vera-whole-health-achieves-validation-endorsement-by-care-innovations-validation-institute-300598404.html.

105 "Pennsylvania Rural Health Model." Centers for Medicare & Medicaid Services, accessed March 20, 2018, https://innovation.cms.gov/initiatives/pa-rural-health-model/.

106 Chase, Dave. "The Best Health Benefits Will Keep the Best Employees in Your Ranks." *HR Daily Advisor,* December 14, 2018. https://hrdailyadvisor.blr.com/2018/12/26/the-best-health-benefits-will-keep-the- best-employees-in-your-ranks/.

107 Chase, Dave. "Why Your Wellness Program Isn't Working - and How to Fix It." US | *Glassdoor for Employers,* January 5, 2019. https://www.glassdoor.com/employers/blog/wellness-program-isnt-working/.

108 Baker, Mike, and Justin Mayo. "The O.R. Factory | Quantity of Care." *Seattle Times.* The Seattle Times Company, February 10, 2017, https://projects.seattletimes.com/2017/quantity-of-care/hospital/.

109 Kenney, Charles. "Better, Faster, More Affordable." *Seattle Business Magazine,* July 2011. https://www.seattlebusinessmag.com/article/better-faster-more-affordable.

110   Chase, Dave. "How to Save Money and Offer Employees Better Coverage with Self-Insurance." *TalentCulture*, April 22, 2019. https://talentculture.com/how-to-save-money-and-offer-employees-better-coverage-with-self-insurance/.

111   "NICE Satmetrix 2018 Consumer Net Promoter Benchmark Study." NICE. NICE, Satmetrix, 2018. http://info.nice.com/rs/338-EJP-431/images/NICE-Satmetrix-infographic-2018-b2c-nps-benchmarks-050418.pdf.

112   "Health Rosetta vs. Status Quo." Health Rosetta. Accessed December 18, 2019. https://healthrosetta.org/learn/health-rosetta-vs-status- quo/.

113   "The Future Health Ecosystem Today," Cascadia Capital, accessed January 15, 2016, http://www.cascadiacapital.com/story/cascadias- digital-healt-care-team-releases-the-future-of-health care-today-report/.

114   "The Future Health Ecosystem Today," Cascadia Capital, accessed January 15, 2016, http://www.cascadiacapital.com/story/cascadias- digital-healt-care-team-releases-the-future-of-health care-today-report/.

115   Dunham, Nancy. "Self-Funded Insurance Cuts Dealer's Costs." *Automotive News*, January 14, 2019. https://www.autonews.com/best-practices/self-funded-insurance-cuts-dealers-costs.

116   Levey, Noam. "Health Insurance Deductibles Soar, Leaving Americans with Unaffordable Bills." *Los Angeles Times*, May 2, 2019.

117   "Fear, Uncertainty, and Doubt." Wikipedia. Wikimedia Foundation, December 17, 2019. https://en.wikipedia.org/wiki/Fear,_uncertainty,_and_doubt.

118   "IOM Report: Estimated $750B Wasted Annually In Health Care System." *Kaiser Health News*, September 7, 2012. https://khn.org/morning-breakout/iom-report/.

119   "The Price of Excess* Identifying Waste in Healthcare Spending." PricewaterhouseCoopers' Health Research Institute. PricewaterhouseCoopers, 2008. http://www.oss.net/dynamaster/file_archive/080509/59f26a38c114f2295757bb6be522128a/The Price of Excess - Identifying Waste in Healthcare Spending - PWC.pdf.

120   Chase, Dave. "Chapter 8: PPO Networks Deliver Value – and Other Flawed Assumptions that Crush Your Budget." *The Opioid Crisis Wake-Up Call*, 85–94. Health Rosetta Media, 2018. https://cdn2.hubspot.net/hubfs/481991/Wake-Up%20Call%20Book/Chapters/CHAPTER%208%20-%20PPO%20networks%20crushing%20your%20budget.pdf.

121   Palosky, Craig, and Sue Ducat. "Premiums for Employer-Sponsored Family Health Coverage Rise 5% to Average $19,616; Single Premiums Rise 3% to $6,896." The Henry J. Kaiser Family Foundation, October 3, 2018. https://www.kff.org/health-costs/press-release/employer-sponsored-family-coverage-premiums-rise-5-percent-in-2018/.

122   Roy, Avik. "In 2018, The Average Family Paid More to Hospitals than to the Federal Government in Taxes." *Forbes Magazine*, March 14, 2019. https://www.forbes.com/sites/theapothecary/2019/01/26/in-2018-the-average-family-paid-more-to-hospitals-than-to-the-federal-government-in-taxes/#56afbb163898.

123   Chase, Dave. "Senator Sanders: No, Saving Hospitals Actually Isn't a Solution to Our Broken Healthcare System." Medium. Tincture, July 17, 2019. https://tincture.io/senator-sanders-no-saving-hospitals-actually-isnt-a-solution-to-our-broken-health care-system-de55b9e1e9d7.

124   Andrzejewski, Adam. "Top U.S. 'Non-Profit' Hospitals & CEOs Are Racking Up Huge Profits." Forbes. Forbes Magazine, August 13, 2019. https://www.forbes.com/sites/adamandrzejewski/2019/06/26/top-u-s-non-profit-hospitals-ceos-are-racking-up-huge-profits/#79087ab19dfb.

125   Hoffman, Reid. "How to Scale a Magical Experience: 4 Lessons from Airbnb's Brian Chesky." *Medium*, May 22, 2018. https://medium.com/@reidhoffman/how-to-scale-a-magical-experience-4-lessons-from-airbnbs-brian-chesky-eca0a182f3e3.

126   Klein, Jeff. "The Four Principles of Conscious Capitalism - Conscious Connection." *Conscious Connection Magazine*, June 20, 2016. https://www.consciousconnectionmagazine.com/2014/05/four-principles-conscious-capitalism/.

127   Chase, Dave. "Economic Development 3.0: Playing the Health Card." LinkedIn. Accessed December 18, 2019. https://www.linkedin.com/pulse/economic-development-30-playing-health-card-dave-chase/.

128   Chase, Dave. "DIY Health Reform from Massachusetts to Alaska." *Forbes*, April 8, 2013. https://www.forbes.com/sites/davechase/2012/03/29/diy-health-reform-from-massachusetts-to-alaska/#3a801897270b.

129   "Charting the Way to Greater Success: Pursuing Perfection in Sweden." Institute for Healthcare Improvement. Accessed December 18, 2019. http://www.ihi.org/resources/Pages/ImprovementStories/ChartingtheWaytoGreaterSuccessPursuingPerfectioninSweden.aspx.

130 Sloane, Sharon. "Why Companies Are Driving Social Change." *Newsweek*, March 27, 2016. https://www.newsweek.com/why-companies-are-driving-social-change-327258.

131 Chase, Dave. "Case Study Rosen Hotels & Resorts." *The Opioid Crisis Wake-Up Call*, 85–94. Health Rosetta Media, 2018. https://cdn2.hubspot.net/hubfs/481991/Wake-Up%20Call%20Book/Case%20Studies/Case%20Study%20Rosen%20Hotels%20&%20Resorts.pdf.

132 Klass, Perri. "Doctors, Is It O.K. If We Talk About Why Finger-Wagging Isn't Working?" *New York Times*, May 6, 2019. https://www.nytimes.com/2019/05/06/well/family/doctors-is-it-ok-if-we-talk-about-why-finger-wagging-isnt-working.html?smid=nytcore-ios-share.

133 "The 8-Step Process for Leading Change: Dr. John Kotter." Kotter. Accessed December 18, 2019. https://www.kotterinc.com/8-steps-process-for-leading-change/.

134 Batshalom, Barbra. "Putting the Management Back in Change Part 5: Removing Obstacles; Empowering Others to Act." Sustainable Performance Institute, October 19, 2019. https://www.sustain-able-performance.org/putting-the-management-back-in-change-part-5-removing-obstacles-empowering-others-to-act/.

INDEX

Index

Made in the USA
Coppell, TX
29 October 2020

40439233R00203